HEALING A FRIEND OR LOVED ONE'S GRIEVING HEART AFTER A CANCER DIAGNOSIS

Also by Alan Wolfelt and Kirby Duvall:

*Healing Your Grieving Heart
After a Cancer Diagnosis:
100 Practical Ideas for Coping,
Surviving, and Thriving*

*Healing Your Grieving Body:
100 Physical Practices for Mourners*

*Healing After Job Loss:
100 Practical Ideas*

Also by Alan Wolfelt:

*Healing Your Grieving Heart:
100 Practical Ideas*

*The Journey Through Grief:
Reflections on Healing*

*The Mourner's Book of Hope:
30 Days of Inspiration*

*Understanding Your Grief:
Ten Essential Touchstones for Finding
Hope and Healing Your Heart*

*Companion Press is dedicated to the education and
support of both the bereaved and bereavement caregivers.
We believe that those who companion the bereaved by
walking with them as they journey in grief have a
wondrous opportunity: to help others embrace and grow
through grief—and to lead fuller, more deeply-lived lives
themselves because of this important ministry.*

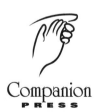

Companion
P R E S S

For a complete catalog and ordering information, write, call, or visit:

Companion Press
The Center for Loss and Life Transition
3735 Broken Bow Road
Fort Collins, CO 80526
(970) 226-6050
www.centerforloss.com

HEALING A FRIEND OR LOVED ONE'S GRIEVING HEART AFTER A CANCER DIAGNOSIS

•

100 PRACTICAL IDEAS FOR PROVIDING COMPASSION, COMFORT, AND CARE

•

ALAN D. WOLFELT, PH.D.
KIRBY J. DUVALL, M.D.

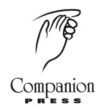

Companion
PRESS

An imprint of the Center for Loss and Life Transition
Fort Collins, Colorado

Companion Press is an imprint of the
Center for Loss and Life Transition
3735 Broken Bow Road
Fort Collins, Colorado 80526
970-226-6050

Companion Press titles may be purchased in bulk for sales
promotions, premiums, or fundraisers. Please contact the
publisher at the above address for more information.

Printed in the United States of America

21 20 19 18 17 16 15 14   5 4 3 2 1

ISBN: 978-1-61722-203-0

In Gratitude

To the families and loved ones of those impacted by cancer who have been willing to share their journeys with us and inspired us to pen this resource.

CONTENTS

INTRODUCTION

Thank you for picking up this book. You probably have it in your hands because someone you care about has been diagnosed with some form of cancer. We want you to know that we're sorry. We offer our sincere empathy to both you and your family member or friend.

While half of all men and one-third of all women in the United States will develop cancer during their lifetimes, it's different when cancer hits close to home. Only then do we become fully aware of the reality of cancer and the many losses it creates.

We wish you courage, grace, comfort, and hope as you begin to explore this resource. Please view this little book as a helper to you in your quest to support the person who has cancer. We hope it inspires in you the strength and empathy to be the cancer companion your family member or friend needs throughout the cancer journey.

My personal story

I was riding my bike in the gorgeous mountains outside of Aspen, Colorado. The day was bright and beautiful. I was enjoying spending the day with my precious daughter Megan and two of her close friends. The furthest thing from my head and heart was anything related to cancer.

Just as I was rounding a slight bend on the bike trail, my cell phone rang. Despite taking a day off for renewal, I had some instinct to answer the call. The female voice on the other end of the line did not mince words. "Is this Dr. Wolfelt?" she asked matter-of-factly. "Yes, it is," I responded. She quickly proceeded. "I'm sorry to have to tell you this on the telephone, but your biopsy results came back, and you have prostate cancer."

I could not move. I could not bring myself to utter even a word in response to her statement. Upon reflection, I don't think I *wanted* the word "cancer" to register with me. My initial response was anchored in a combination of shock, fear, and protest. I don't remember any words that passed between us after I heard those dreaded words, "You have cancer."

When the shock evolved to overwhelming sadness, I began to think about how I didn't want to leave my wife, Sue, and my three beloved children, Megan, Chris, and Jaimie. I said to myself, "Is this it? Am I going to die in my 50s? What if I don't survive this? I have so much to live for—more love to give, more books to write, more workshops to teach. I'm not ready to go!" This was the start of my rollercoaster ride of self-examination and personal discovery.

Not only am I a cancer survivor, I am a grief counselor and educator. For more than thirty years, I have taught people about the need to embrace and express their grief after a significant loss so they can go on to live and love well again. Central to this mission has also been the education of caregivers who have the privilege of helping others affected by grief and loss. This book, then, sits squarely at the intersection of two important pieces of my life.

Cancer is loss

For your friend or family member as well as for all those who care about someone with cancer, cancer is a significant loss.

No matter your friend's type or stage of cancer or survivorship, his life changed after his diagnosis. From the moment he first heard those three little words, he experienced losses of many kinds.

He lost his health. Even if he recovered his health in the months and years after his treatment, he knows what it means to feel healthy one moment and frighteningly unhealthy the next. He also lost his sense of normalcy and safety. He may have lost his ability to work and his financial stability. In the course of his treatment, perhaps he lost a body part or two, his hair, his appetite, his memory (thanks to chemo brain), and even some of his friends. (Not everyone is capable of the steadfastness it takes to be a companion through the cancer journey. More on that in a moment.)

You are probably all too aware that the friends and family members of the person with cancer experience myriad losses as well. Your sense of normalcy and safety has also been threatened. You begin to consider and grieve the worst-case scenarios. Depending on your relationship with the person who has cancer and the activities you share, you may have, at least temporarily, lost your golf partner, your walking buddy, or even your lover. In general, you have probably lost the easy enjoyment of spending time with this person.

So yes, in many ways, cancer is synonymous with loss. And when we lose things (or people) that we care about or that are important to our sense of self, we naturally grieve.

Grief and mourning

Grief is what we think and feel on the inside when we lose someone or something important. When someone we love is diagnosed with a life-threatening illness, we experience shock, anger, guilt, sadness, and other emotions. We think many dark and difficult thoughts. All of these thoughts and feelings go into a pot called grief.

Mourning is the word for grief expressed. While grief is what's bottled up inside you, mourning is the opening up, the letting out, and the sharing.

Without mourning, grief festers. Contrary to the cliché "time heals all wounds," grief does not magically dissipate through the passage of time alone. If it is not expressed fully and honestly, it tends to result in ongoing problems such as depression, intimacy troubles, chronic anxiety, substance abuse, and others.

But *with* mourning? Oh, with mourning, what amazing rewards await us on the far side of grief! When genuinely expressed, grief has the potential to open us to a richer and deeper experience of life.

Both you and your friend or family member will naturally grieve in the weeks and months after the diagnosis. This book provides encouragement and ideas intended to help both of you mourn.

Being a cancer companion

If you are reading this book, you surely have the intention to be a good helper during the cancer journey. That's a good start. Intention is where everything begins.

Now to your intention you must add *action*. You must reach out and keep reaching out to the person who has cancer. You must offer your presence and your empathy for the long haul. You must persevere long after most friends and even family members fall away.

You see, not everyone has the endurance to be a good helper for months and years, which is often how long the cancer journey takes. Yet this is exactly what the person who has cancer needs most—people she can count on, well, forever.

Throughout this book you will notice that I use the term "cancer companion" to describe your role in helping your friend or family member. When broken down into its original Latin roots, the word "companion" means *com* for "with" and *pan* for "bread"—in other words, someone you would share a meal with. This is how I want you to think about being a good friend or family member through the wilderness of cancer. Cancer companions spend time with the people they care about who have cancer. They share meals sometimes, yes, but they also have conversations. Importantly, they listen. They have empathy. They are sounding boards and, sometimes, whipping posts.

Cancer companions accompany people with cancer on their journeys. They do not walk in front of or behind the person with cancer. They walk alongside, arm-in-arm. And they continue to offer their presence and loving companionship as long as the journey lasts.

If the person with cancer is someone you deeply love

This book is entitled *Healing A Friend or Loved One's Grieving Heart After A Cancer Diagnosis*, but the word "friend" encompasses many different kinds of relationships and degrees of closeness. Also, I realize you might be reading this book if you are a family member of the person with cancer.

Regardless of the label our culture might place on your relationship, the bottom line is that the more connected you feel to the person who has cancer, the more you, too, will struggle with the diagnosis and grieve throughout her cancer journey. Also, the closer you are to the person with cancer, the more help you will need for yourself in the coming weeks and months.

Because of your normal and necessary grief, you may find it impossible to be as supportive of the person who has cancer as you would like to be. That's how grief works. But if you get good support for yourself and work on expressing all your fears, thoughts, and feelings (by sharing them with the person with cancer but also in other ways, such as journaling or attending a support group), you will be better able to help the person with cancer. You will also find hope and healing for yourself.

(A caution: Take care not to over-share your own fears and anxieties about the person's cancer. Don't lie to him or feign rosy thoughts, but do be respectful of the timing and pacing of sharing your true concerns. If he is projecting feelings of shock or denial, he might not be ready to talk about worst cancer fears. As always, let him take the lead. When he is ready to share his fears, that is probably a good time for you to share yours as well. In the meantime, do talk about and express any fears you may have to someone else.)

Throughout this book we will use the terms friend and family member more or less interchangeably. Please know that whatever your relationship to the person who has cancer, we are thinking of you and very much include you in our suggestions.

How to use this book

I wrote this book together with my longtime friend and physician Dr. Kirby Duvall. To my passion about helping others in grief and my own cancer survivorship, he adds decades of medical experience helping patients during and after their treatment for cancer. While this is more of a spiritual guide to cancer than a medical one, his medical expertise informs a number of the ideas you'll find here.

As promised, this book contains 100 ideas to help you provide compassion, comfort, and care to your friend or family member who has cancer. Some of the ideas will teach you about the basic principles of grief, mourning, empathy, and cancer companionship. The remainder offer practical, here-and-now, action-oriented suggestions for helping the person who has cancer. Each idea is followed by a brief explanation of how and why the idea might be useful.

Some of the ideas will speak to your unique circumstances better than others. If you come to an idea that doesn't seem to fit, simply ignore it and turn to another page.

As you flip through these pages, you will also see that each idea includes a "Carpe Diem," which means, as fans of the movie *Dead Poets Society* will remember, "seize the day." Our hope is that you not relegate this resource to your shelves but instead keep it handy on your nightstand or desk. Pick it up often and turn to any page; the Carpe Diem suggestion might help you seize the day by giving you a cancer companionship exercise, action, or thought to consider today, right now, right this minute.

Please understand that nothing is this book should be construed as medical advice. If you have questions or concerns about any medical matter, you should consult your doctor or other healthcare provider. You should never delay seeking medical advice, disregard medical advice, or discontinue medical treatment (or advise any of those things to your friend or family member) because of information contained in this book.

We thank you for taking the time to read and reflect on the words that make up this book. We wish you courage and grace as you companion the person you care about on the cancer journey.

Godspeed. We hope to meet you one day.

Alan D. Wolfelt

1.

UNDERSTAND WHAT CANCER IS

"Growth for the sake of growth is the ideology of the cancer cell."
— Edward Abbey

- Our bodies make new cells all the time so that we can grow, heal ourselves when we've been hurt, and replace worn-out cells. Every day, our bodies make perfect cells as well as imperfect ones. Fortunately, imperfect cells usually either die or are unable to divide and multiply. Our bodies have cellular quality control built in.

- But sometimes, abnormal cells find ways to divide and multiply without control. The cells form colonies called tumors (except blood cancers, which act differently). Some of the abnormal cells can sneak into the bloodstream or the lymphatic system and migrate to other places in the body. This is called *metastasis*, and when it happens, tumors begin to form throughout the body.

- Tumors interfere with the necessary functions of our bodies' organs and blood vessels. As they invade and grow, they cut off oxygen, obstruct the GI system, and create openings there there aren't supposed to be openings.

- There are more than 100 kinds of cancer. We name cancers by the place where they start. Breast cancer begins in the breast, for example. If it spreads to the brain, it is still breast cancer. Pathologists can tell where a cancer originated by looking at the cells under a microscope.

- Cancers are said to have "stages." Staging describes the extent or severity of a person's cancer. Knowing the stage helps doctors and other caregivers choose the best treatment. It also conveys a probable prognosis. Cancer staging ranges from zero to IV (zero, I, II, III, and IV), with zero being the least serious and IV the most.

CARPE DIEM

Learn a little more about your friend's cancer today—not to scare you but to help you be more conversant and supportive. The National Cancer Institute's website, www.cancer.gov, is a good resource.

2.

UNDERSTAND HOW CANCER IS TREATED

"Chemotherapy is brutal. The goal is pretty much to kill everything in your body without killing you."

— Rashida Jones

- There are three main forms of cancer treatment:
  1. Surgery—The tumor (or as much of it as possible) is removed. For operable tumors, this is usually the first step in treatment. Lymph nodes near the tumor may also be removed to see if they have been invaded by cancer cells. If the entire tumor can be removed and the lymph nodes are clear, surgery may be the only treatment required.
  2. Chemotherapy—Drugs that destroy cancer cells are taken either by mouth or intravenously. They attack rapidly dividing cells in the body, which includes cancer cells as well as some healthy cells. It is the harming of healthy cells that makes some cancer patients feel sick and experience other unpleasant side effects (such as hair loss).
  3. Radiation—Strong beams of energy are targeted directly at the tumor, killing or shrinking it. Patients may receive radiation therapy before, during, or after surgery. Often patients receive radiation in small doses every day for several weeks. Some patients receive only radiation therapy, while others receive radiation as well as chemotherapy.
- Your friend may need different kinds of help during and after different kinds of treatment. If he is receiving radiation therapy, for example, he may need someone to accompany him to the radiation oncologist's office every day for half an hour. During chemotherapy, he may prefer help with housework. Ask.

CARPE DIEM
During treatment, be on the watch for help your friend needs most. Offer. Be specific.

3.

UNDERSTAND THE DIFFERENCE BETWEEN GRIEF AND MOURNING

"What happens when people open their hearts? They get better."
— Haruki Murakami

• Grief is the constellation of internal thoughts and feelings we experience when we lose something or someone we care about—or when we are threatened with the possibility of such a loss. Grief is the weight in the chest, the churning in the gut, the unspeakable thoughts and feelings.

• Mourning is the outward expression of our grief. Mourning is crying, journaling, creating artwork, talking to others, telling the story, speaking the unspeakable.

• Here's a way to remember which is which: The "i" in grief stands for what I feel inside. The "u" in mourn reminds me to share my grief with you.

• Everyone grieves when they are affected by life's challenges, but if we are to heal emotionally and spiritually, we must also mourn. Over time, and with the support of others, to mourn is to heal.

• Many of the ideas in this book are intended to help you mourn the natural and necessary grief that is a result of caring about someone who has cancer. Others are directed at helping you become a more empathetic cancer companion—someone who supports the person with cancer as she expresses her own natural and necessary grief.

CARPE DIEM
Ask yourself this question: Have I been mourning my friend's cancer, or have I mostly been restricting myself to grieving?

4.

ALLOW FOR NUMBNESS

"There is a feeling of disbelief that comes over you, that takes over, and you kind of go through the motions. You do what you're supposed to do, but in fact you're not there at all."

— Frederick Barthelme

• Did you feel numb and in shock in the days and weeks right after your loved one's cancer diagnosis? It's very common to feel blindsided by the news that someone you care about has a life-threatening illness.

• Feelings of shock, numbness, and disbelief are nature's way of temporarily protecting us from the full force of a painful reality. Like anesthesia, these feelings help us survive the pain of our early grief. Be thankful for numbness.

• We often think, "I will wake up and this will not have happened." Early grief can feel like being in a dream. Your emotions need time to catch up with what your mind has been told.

• Soon you will come to understand the diagnosis and prognosis intellectually, with your head. Only over time will you come to understand them with your heart.

• Of course, your friend will also experience his own days and weeks of shock, numbness, and even denial. You can affirm that these feelings are normal. You can also help by stepping in to coordinate appointments, prescriptions, groceries, etc. when the person you care about is too numb or shocked to be thinking clearly.

CARPE DIEM

If you're feeling numb and distracted by news of your friend's cancer, take it easy for a few days. Cancel any commitments that aren't absolutely necessary.

5.

HELP YOUR FRIEND FOCUS ON FIRST THINGS FIRST

"What happens when my body breaks down happens not just to that body but also to my life, which is lived in that body. When the body breaks down, so does the life."

— Arthur Frank

• Have you ever seen the psychologist Abraham Maslow's famous "hierarchy of needs"? It's a pyramid that shows the natural and normal priority of human needs.

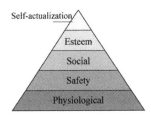

• The base of the pyramid is formed by our physiological needs—in other words, the needs of our bodies. If your friend is in the middle of treatment right now, his body is under attack and will likely demand all his attention for a while. He needs to get ample rest, eat as well as he can, stay hydrated, and get relief from any pain he might be experiencing.

• Until his needs for physical comfort and safety are met, he simply can't move up the pyramid to address his other needs.

• Help your friend focus on first things first. Make sure she is being taken good care of physically. Only if she is feeling well enough will she be able to engage emotionally and socially with the people who care about her and with her own spirit.

• Of course, Maslow's hierarchy of needs applies to you, too! You can't support your friend with cancer socially and emotionally unless you first take care of your own body's needs. Don't make the mistake of thinking you can ignore the bottom of *your* pyramid, because if you do, your own life may come crashing down.

CARPE DIEM

Ask yourself: How am I feeling physically right now, this very minute? Am I tired? Hungry? Stiff? In pain? Attend to your physical needs immediately.

6.

DON'T SAY THIS

"Attempting to get at truth means rejecting stereotypes and clichés."
— Harold Evans

- Most of us are guilty of offering clichés and platitudes when talking to someone who is experiencing challenges and loss. But now that you're reading this book, it's time to stop.
- In a well-intentioned (but misguided) effort to talk to someone about her cancer, you might say…
    - I know how you feel.
    - So-and-so had _____ cancer, too.
    - It's all part of God's plan.
    - God works in mysterious ways.
    - God only gives you what you can handle.
    - But you look perfectly healthy!
    - Why didn't you tell me sooner?
    - You'll beat this. I know you will.
    - Everything is going to be just fine.
    - You just need to stay positive.
- Do you notice how none of these remarks are focused on the unique and particular experiences, thoughts, and feelings of the person with cancer? Instead, they are either about you or about providing impossibly simple answers to exceptionally complex problems.
- If you feel a cliché forming on your lips, bite your tongue. Say something from Idea 7 instead.

CARPE DIEM
Right now, commit several of the responses in Idea 7 to memory.

7.

DO SAY THIS

"Once someone said to me, 'I'll ride the waves with you till the storm calms,' and that meant a lot to me because I knew they would be with me no matter what."

— Author Unknown

- I'm sorry you have to go through this.
- I want you to know I care about you.
- How can I help? I'm good at _____,
  _____, and _____.
- How are you doing? I want to know.
- Would you like to talk about it? I would like to be someone you can talk to.
- I don't know what to say, but I feel love and concern for you.
- I'm going to the store today. What can I get for you?
- I don't know what that diagnosis means. Would you mind telling me what it means for you?
- What do you most need help with?
- I was thinking about you today, so I called (or stopped by).
- You are important to me.
- You are a very special person to me.
- I love you.

CARPE DIEM
Today, reach out to the person with cancer and tell her one of these things. Then listen.

8.

DEVELOP THE ART OF EMPATHY

*"When we honestly ask ourselves which people in our lives mean the
most to us, we often find it is those who, instead of giving advice,
solutions, or cures, have chosen rather to share our pain and touch our
wounds with a warm and tender hand."*

— Henri Nouwen

- The words "sympathy" and "empathy" are often used interchangeably, yet there is an important difference between the two—a difference you can leverage to make yourself a better helper.

- When you are sympathetic to someone else, you are noticing and feeling concern for his circumstances, usually at a distance. You are "feeling sorry" for him. You are feeling "pity" for him. You are looking at his situation from the outside, and you are acknowledging the distress passively. You may be offering a simple solution, platitude, or distraction. Sometimes sympathy also includes a touch (or a heavy dose) of judgment or superiority. Sympathy is "feeling for" someone else.

- Empathy, on the other hand, is about making an emotional connection. It is a more active process—one in which you try to understand and feel the other person's experience from the inside out. You are not judging the person or the circumstances. You are not offering solutions. Instead, you are making yourself vulnerable to the person's thoughts, feelings, and circumstances by looking for connections to similar thoughts, feelings, and circumstances inside you. You are being present and allowing yourself to be taught by the other person. Empathy is "feeling with" someone else.

- If you feel sympathy for the person with cancer but want to *do something* about it, you are experiencing an urge to be more empathetic. Be brave and steadfast enough to follow this urge where it leads.

CARPE DIEM

Today, convert your sympathy for someone into active empathy and
see what happens.

9.

UNDERSTAND THE SIX
NEEDS OF MOURNING

**Need #1: Acknowledge the reality of your friend's diagnosis
and prognosis**

*"You hear the word 'cancer' and you think it is a death sentence. In
fact, the shock is the biggest thing about a diagnosis of cancer."*

— Clare Balding

- Someone you care about has cancer. This may be a difficult reality
for you to accept. Yet gently, slowly, and patiently, you must embrace
this reality, bit by bit, day by day.

- Growing comfortable with speaking the words aloud may help
you with this mourning need. Learning to say, "My friend has
_____ cancer" to other friends and family members when
the need arises will help you come to terms with the reality of his
diagnosis and prognosis.

- At times you may push away the reality of your friend's cancer,
especially if the prognosis is grim. This is normal and necessary for
your survival. You will come to integrate the reality in doses as you
are ready.

- Of course, each of the six needs of mourning applies to your friend's
cancer journey as well. You can help her with Need #1 by listening
as she talks about her diagnosis and prognosis and reflecting back
what she tells you. Trying to soothe her with unrealistic clichés (e.g.,
"You'll be fine!") runs counter to this need and is not helpful.

CARPE DIEM
Maybe you've been keeping this reality from someone in your own life.
Today, tell this person.

10.

UNDERSTAND THE SIX
NEEDS OF MOURNING

Need #2: Embrace the pain of your losses

*"In the godforsaken, obscene quicksand of life, there is a deafening
alleluia rising from the souls of those who weep, and of those who weep
with those who weep. If you watch, you will see the hand of God
putting the stars back in their skies one by one."*

— Ann Weems

- This need requires people in grief to embrace the pain of their
  losses—something we naturally don't want to do. It is easier to avoid,
  repress, or push away the pain than it is to confront it.

- It is in embracing your grief, however, that you will learn to reconcile
  yourself to it.

- In the early days after your friend's diagnosis, you may feel the hurt
  often, especially if you have a close relationship with this person.
  During this time, you will probably need to seek refuge from your
  pain now and then. Go for a walk, read a book, watch TV, talk to
  supportive friends and family about the normal things of everyday
  life.

- In small doses and over time, your friend must also embrace the pain
  of having his life affected by—and perhaps cut short by—cancer. You
  can help by being a reliable listener and continued presence in his
  life.

CARPE DIEM
Today, talk to someone else about the painful thoughts and feelings
you are experiencing as a result of your friend's cancer.

11.

UNDERSTAND THE SIX NEEDS OF MOURNING

Need #3: Remember your past

"Memory is a way of holding onto the things you love, the things you are, the things you never want to lose."
— Kevin Arnold

- We often say that remembering the past makes hoping for the future possible.
- Life is so hectic today that we rarely take time to revel in precious memories and old loves and friendships. We are so busy doing that we don't have time just "being."
- Cancer is a wake-up call—both to the person with cancer and to all those who care about her.
- You will probably find yourself instinctively returning to memories of special times you've shared with the person who has cancer. (That's because remembering your past is a mourning need!) When we as humans experience threats to our safety or relationships, we instinctively go backward. When you have these urges and moments of remembering, take the time to slow down and really explore them.
- Your friend will also experience this mourning need. You can help by reminiscing with him, encouraging him to share memories with you, and looking at old photos and videos together.

CARPE DIEM
Today, make it a point to recount a special memory with the person who has cancer.

12.

UNDERSTAND THE SIX
NEEDS OF MOURNING

Need #4: Incorporate cancer into your life story

"People's view of cancer will change when they have their own relationship with cancer, which everyone will, at some point."

— Laura Linney

- Someone you care about has cancer. Coming to terms with the fact that your life has been touched by cancer is one of your needs of mourning.

- Until it happens to us or to someone we love, cancer seems like one of those things that happens to other people. But now cancer has become part of your life's journey.

- The first time someone you care about is diagnosed with cancer, it can feel like entering a room that you've never been inside before. You knew the room existed, but you didn't know quite what it would be like—and you didn't want to ever step inside. But here you are, in the cancer room, probably with lots of other people you know. What does it feel like to be there? Talking to other friends and family members affected by cancer will help you work on this mourning need.

- You can help your friend work on this need of mourning by listening without judgment as she struggles to incorporate cancer and its ongoing challenges into her own self-identity.

CARPE DIEM

Write out a response to this prompt: I used to feel _____ about cancer. Since my friend's cancer diagnosis, I feel _____. What's different is that _____.
Keep writing as long as you want.

13.

UNDERSTAND THE SIX
NEEDS OF MOURNING

Need #5: Search for meaning

*"Because there is no glory in illness. There is no meaning to it. There is
no honor in dying of it."*

— John Green

- When someone we care about is diagnosed with a life-threatening illness, we naturally question the meaning and purpose of life and death.
- "Why" questions may surface uncontrollably and often precede "How" questions. "Why did this have to happen?" and "Why my friend?" come before "How will I go on if she dies?"
- Sometimes we are taught, "Don't ask why. It doesn't do you any good." Yet it is natural to ask why and search for meaning in the face of cancer.
- You will almost certainly question your philosophy of life and explore religious and spiritual values as you work on this need. So will your friend. This is normal and natural.
- Remember that having faith or spirituality does not negate your need to mourn. Even if you believe in an afterlife of some kind, both your friend's life and your life here on Earth have still been affected by cancer. It's normal to feel dumbfounded and angry at a God whom you may feel has permitted such a thing to happen.
- Ultimately, you may decide that there is no answer to the question "Why did this happen?" Allow your friend to explore such questions without trying to provide an answer.

CARPE DIEM
Write down a list of "Why" questions that have surfaced for you since your friend's diagnosis. Find another friend to talk to who will explore these questions with you without thinking she has to give you answers.

14.

UNDERSTAND THE SIX
NEEDS OF MOURNING

Need #6: Receive ongoing support from others

"When someone has cancer, the whole family and everyone who loves them does, too."

— Terri Clark

- As mourners, we need the love and understanding of others if we are to heal. This goes for you as well as for the person with cancer.
- Unfortunately, our society places too much value on "carrying on" and "doing well." Don't be surprised if others forget that you are struggling with the cancer journey of someone you care about. And keep in mind that it's common for many friends and family members to stop supporting the person with cancer herself after the first few weeks.
- For you, other people whose lives have been closely touched by cancer may be an excellent source of social, emotional, and spiritual support. They "get it." Consider joining a support group.
- Grief is experienced in "doses" over months and years, not quickly and efficiently, and you may need the continued support of your friends and family for a long time. Of course, your friend with cancer also needs long-term support. Every time I (Alan) return to my oncologist's office for a routine PSA check, my anxiety goes up. I appreciate my friends and family members who listen and support me as I express my anxiety.

CARPE DIEM
Look into support groups for cancer companions.

15.

HELP HER LEARN TO ACCEPT HELP

"I am because we are."
— African Proverb

• One of your friend's mourning needs is to receive and accept help from others. Neither cancer nor grief is a do-it-yourself activity. But not everyone is a good "helpee." Some people feel shame or embarrassment over not being able to handle things themselves. Others have always been the givers or helpers and have a hard time when tables are turned.

• You can be the cancer companion who steps in and says to your friend, "You need help right now. I'm here to help you. Others want to help, too. Please let us. We love you."

• If your friend shrugs off attempts to help her, don't take "no" for an answer. Try your best to help her anyway. Tell her that *you* need to help *her*—even if in very small ways.

• We're not advocating codependency here. Sometimes people with cancer want and need to feel normal and capable. Don't take this away from them. But do look for opportunities when they really and truly *do* need help. These are the times when you may need to supportively confront them about rebuffing the love and attention of others.

CARPE DIEM
If your friend insists that she doesn't need help, remind her of a time when she helped you or someone else. Tell her it's her turn to be taken care of now.

16.

SHOW UP

"Mouths closed. Ears open. Presence available."
— Author Unknown

- The best way to help someone who is undergoing cancer diagnosis and treatment (and its aftermath) is to simply be there.
- Cancer is often an isolating experience. It's common for people with cancer to feel at once surrounded by doctors, nurses, and other cancer patients yet at the same time very alone. Life-threatening illness naturally pulls people inward. It forces them to confront their deepest feelings and beliefs and their own mortality in very interior ways. This internal struggle can be challenging, if not impossible, to fully share with others. And because treatment can last a long time, friends and family who were initially helpful and "there" for the person with cancer tend to fall away over the many weeks and months.
- Don't assume that your friend with cancer has lots of other friends and family members actively helping him. This is often an illusion. While I (Alan) knew that my family was very concerned about me, I still felt very alone on the day of my surgery and in the weeks that followed.
- Regardless of how many others the person with cancer has in her life, you can choose to be someone who consistently shows up—for months and years.
- Call. E-mail. Text. Send cards. Skype. And most important and whenever possible, be there in person, face-to-face. Read Ideas 17 and 18 for more on "being there."

CARPE DIEM
Today, if at all possible, spend an hour or more with the person who has cancer.

17.

BE A GREAT LISTENER

"Most people do not listen with the intent to understand. They listen with the intent to reply."
— Stephen R. Covey

- The person with cancer is hurting inside. She may be hurting physically and is almost certainly hurting emotionally, socially, cognitively, and spiritually. In other words, she is grieving. While you can't take her pain away, you can listen as she shares her painful thoughts and feelings.

- Being a good listener to someone with cancer means listening without judging or trying to take his feelings away. It means empathizing and being present to the pain. It does not mean trying to fix things, give easy answers, or stop the tears. Often it means listening and not saying anything in return.

- Lean in, make eye contact, offer touch when appropriate, and listen.

- On the other hand, some people aren't talkers. They're not used to or good at openly expressing their inner thoughts and feelings. How do you "listen" to these silent types? By simply spending time with them. While you're playing cards, watching a movie, or folding laundry together, communication will naturally happen—verbally or nonverbally. One way or another, if you are consistently present to her, the person with cancer will share her thoughts and feelings in dribs and drabs. And it is your presence that will make her essential mourning possible.

CARPE DIEM
Pick an opportunity to work on your active listening skills today.

18.

BE PRESENT

"We can live forever, a minute at a time."
— Author Unknown

• In our world of constant technological connectivity, it's easier than ever to stay in touch with the news, with pop-culture happenings, with far-flung friends and family, and with our closest loved ones, too. As technology becomes more pervasive, though, it's getting harder and harder to be truly present to those we love.

• Being present means looking and listening without distraction. It means attending to someone else fully and exclusively. It can also mean really experiencing something alongside or together with someone else.

• Being present to the person with cancer means putting your cell phone, tablet, and laptop away while you are with him. It means focusing on him and offering him your full attention if he wants it. If you are accompanying him to the doctor's office or to the grocery store or to the beach, it means putting his needs first and making sure he is comfortable and well cared for. It means allowing his needs to guide the discussion and activities.

• More and more, being present is an art that few of us practice. Yet, ironically, presence is where truth, beauty, and love reside.

CARPE DIEM

Today, spend one hour being fully present to the person with cancer or to someone else you love.

19.

PRACTICE PATIENCE

"Why is patience so important?"
"Because it makes us pay attention."
— Paulo Coelho

- You may have realized by now that the cancer journey is often long and uncertain. And because your friend's cancer experience becomes part of who she is, and by extension, part of who you are, it never really, totally, ever goes away.

- In our hurry-up North American culture, patience can be especially hard to come by. We have all been conditioned to believe that if we want something, we should be able to get it instantly. But cancer diagnosis and treatment doesn't work like that. And cancer itself usually doesn't respond like that.

- And so, you must practice patience. Be patient with yourself. Be patient with your friend who has cancer. Be patient with his other friends and his family. Be patient with your friends and family. Most of the time, everyone is doing the best they can (even when it seems like they're not).

- Practicing patience means relinquishing control, too. Although you would certainly make her PET scans 100 percent clear if you could, you cannot. Neither she nor you nor her doctors really have control over her illness. Coming to terms with this fact will be part of your journey—and hers as well.

CARPE DIEM
When you are feeling impatient, silently repeat this phrase: I am here. I am now. You are here. You are now. May God bless us both.

20.

OFFER PRACTICAL HELP

"We only have what we give."
— Isabel Allende

- When someone is undergoing cancer treatment, he needs help. Whether he comes right out and says it or not, he's almost certainly struggling with some or many aspects of his life. I (Alan) certainly know I questioned everything about my life: my relationships, my vocation, my God.

- Imagine that taking care of your health was essentially a full-time job right now—AND, in addition to this full-time job, you were feeling really crappy and tired. That's what it may well be like for your friend or family member with cancer.

- Offer emotional support how and when you can, yes, but also offer practical help. Pitch in with errands, meals, and other chores. Help take care of children or pets. Offer to sort through or handle paperwork. What are your skills or strengths? Do that.

- Also, and very importantly, be specific. Don't say, "Let me know if you need anything." Instead, say, "I'd like to bring over dinner one night this week. Which day is best?" or "Would you like to go for a walk this afternoon?" or "I'm going to the grocery store today. What do you need?"

- You may be a natural helper, someone who steps in easily to do what needs doing. But if you're not a natural helper, try being one now. Go outside your comfort zone. Give of yourself. It will help everyone involved, including you.

CARPE DIEM
Do something that needs doing for the person with cancer's immediate family or household without being asked.

21.

GIVE YOUR FRIEND A JOURNAL

"From time to time, I'll look back through the personal journals I've scribbled in throughout my life, the keepers of my raw thoughts and emotions. The words poured forth after my dad died, when I went through a divorce, and after I was diagnosed with breast cancer. There are so many what-ifs scribbled on those pages."

— Hoda Kotb

- Cancer is a journey. So is grief.
- Have you ever noticed how the words "journey" and "journal" are similar? Both come from the French word *jour*, which means "day." As your friend journeys through cancer and grief, one day a time, he may be helped by capturing his daily thoughts, feelings, and experiences in a journal.
- Even if she doesn't think of herself as a "writer," she might want to give it a try now. Journaling is a form of outward expression of her interior reality. It's mourning! And as I've emphasized, mourning is how she moves toward healing her cancer grief and living and loving fully.
- You might also want to try journaling! It's a healing and self-revealing habit.

CARPE DIEM

Pick out a nice journal and pen for your friend today. While you're at it, buy a set for yourself.

22.

HELP WITH APPETITE ISSUES

*"I knew when I was diagnosed with cancer the only thing I could
control was what I ate, what I drank, and what I would think."*

— Kris Carr

• Cancer and its treatment often cause appetite loss and other eating
problems, which can in turn lead to weight loss as well as loss of
strength. Poor appetite may be caused by swallowing problems,
anxiety, depression, pain or nausea, and vomiting. It can also be due
to a change in sense of taste or smell, feeling full, tumor growth,
dehydration, or side effects of chemotherapy or radiation.

• So don't be surprised if your friend doesn't seem to want to eat.
You can help, though, by reminding her that food is a necessary
part of her treatment as well as her wellbeing. (Remember Maslow's
pyramid?) Small, frequent meals composed of her favorite foods are
usually the best bet.

• The quality of the food he eats matters, too, so try to ensure that he's
getting enough protein and antioxidant-rich fruits and vegetables.

• Create a pleasant setting for meals and take the time to eat with your
friend.

CARPE DIEM

Is your friend nauseated? Think ginger. Ginger candies, ginger cookies,
ginger tea, ginger in stir fry, and powdered ginger sprinkled over rice
will help combat nausea.

23.

BE CAREFUL ABOUT SHARING OTHERS' CANCER STORIES OR OFFERING ADVICE

"When I meet people who say, which they do all of the time, 'My great aunt had cancer of the elbow, and the doctors gave her ten seconds to live, but last I heard she was climbing Mount Everest,' and so forth, I switch off quite early."

— Christopher Hitchens

- We all know people whose lives have been touched or devasted by cancer. Maybe you yourself have had cancer.

- In that way, cancer is indeed a shared human experience. But here's the thing: Your friend or family member with cancer is experiencing his own very unique journey. Being told how someone else was miraculously cured or had it worse than him or had the same type of cancer may only serve to make him feel like a failure or a statistic. I (Alan) had several people share these kinds of things with me, and I wanted to get away from them as fast as I could.

- When you start telling "cancer stories," you take the focus off the person you are supposed to be supporting and put it on yourself. Please, don't do this.

- If the person with cancer asks or brings it up, then by all means, share cancer stories or advice. But if she doesn't ask, take her cue and instead focus on empathizing with her unique situation, thoughts, and feelings.

- Sharing cancer stories often works best in the mutually supportive, "we're-in-this-together, right-now" context of a support group. If the person with cancer wants to attend a support group, you can help by researching groups and coordinating transportation.

CARPE DIEM

The next time you have the urge to share a cancer story with the person who has cancer, stop yourself and ask him instead, "What is happening with you right now?"

24.

COME BEARING JOY

"When you do things from your soul, you feel a river moving in you, a joy."
— Rumi

- Cancer is a slog. It can be a long, arduous, painful process. Among diseases, it's often one of the marathons.
- You can be one of the kind people staffing the marathon water stations, only instead of offering water here and there along the way, you'll be offering joy.
- Bring fresh flowers you cut from your yard. Bake her favorite cookies. Rent five great comedies (or check them out from the library) and drop them off at her house. Sit and watch her favorite ballgame with her. Load up an iPod with audiobooks and give it to her. Play an instrument for her. Sing her a song. Tell her a joke.
- If you're a busy person, do double duty. Whenever you do or make something, do it twice and share with him. For example, if you're making lasagna, make two and give one to him. If you're picking up muffins at the bakery, grab some for him, too. If you're sending someone a card, send one to him as well.
- Don't confuse this approach with being a "cheerleader" who is always upbeat and bubbly and who doesn't empathize when the person with cancer is experiencing sadness and dark emotions. Don't be a Tigger. But don't be an Eeyore, either. Instead, strive to mirror and "receive" the emotional-spiritual tone of your friend or family member. And remember that you can still bring flowers or cookies—in other words, bits of joy—on sad days.

CARPE DIEM
Make delivering joy a habit. It just might change your life for the better, too.

25.

BE HER SECRETARY (OR FIND SOMEONE WHO CAN BE)

"If you cannot do great things, do small things in a great way."
— Author Unknown

- After a cancer diagnosis comes a tsunami of medical lingo, treatment information, and complex choices. What's more, the person with cancer is often dealing with multiple doctors and care providers. It can get extremely confusing.

- The person with cancer could probably use some help organizing all this information and paperwork. Wouldn't it be best for him to spend his limited energy on his health and healing?

- Making a cancer notebook is one good technique. It's a place where she can write down questions, physician names and phone numbers, appointment dates and times, prescription information, daily notes on side effects, etc. She can take it to every appointment and keep it handy by the phone.

- You can help get the cancer notebook started. If possible, you can attend appointments with her and take notes. If that's not possible, maybe you can identify someone else who can do it. If you're good at paperwork, you could also help with insurance claims and medical bills.

- Some health systems offer the free services of a "cancer navigator"— usually a nurse whose job is to help patients and families understand and effectively navigate the treatment labyrinth. Find out if there's a navigator in your friend's healthcare system and learn how he can take advantage of it.

CARPE DIEM
Today, find out if the person who has cancer needs help with paperwork, scheduling, or other administrative tasks.

26.

ACCEPT ALL THOUGHTS AND EMOTIONS WITH EQUANIMITY

"To be fully seen by somebody, then, and be loved anyhow—this is a human offering that can border on miraculous."
— Elizabeth Gilbert

- With a diagnosis of cancer come many significant losses. The person you are trying to companion has lost his health, his sense of normalcy and safety, his day-to-day routine. Depending on the course of treatment and prognosis, he may have also lost his job or his financial stability. This is a lot to try to cope with, and it's normal for him to react with a whole range of thoughts and feelings.

- We often say that thoughts and feelings are not right or wrong, they just are. This goes for the person with cancer and as well as you.

- If the person with cancer is having a persistent thought or feeling, that means she needs to express it. It's the expression of her thoughts and feelings that will help her cope and even thrive during her cancer journey. Your job is to listen, without judging, as she shares.

- Is she angry? That's OK. Does she feel guilty? That's OK. Has she had some crazy thoughts? That's OK, too. Try not to tell her that she shouldn't think or feel as she does. Instead, listen and try to empathize with her thoughts and feelings.

- It's hard to actively listen to people expressing difficult emotions, such as rage or despair. As a companion to someone with cancer, your job isn't easy. But if you can be that safe harbor in which he knows he can share *anything*, he'll be sharing his truth and making way for more peace, love, and joy in the days to come.

CARPE DIEM

If you want to get better at accepting the full gamut of thoughts and feelings, ask someone to role-play with you. Have him share some real or pretend difficult emotions. Practice responding with open-ended questions and statements that confirm that you heard and accept him.

27.

EXPECT MOOD SWINGS

"Cancer is not a straight line. It's up and down."
— Elizabeth Edwards

- The cancer journey often has a lot of ups and downs. Your friend's diagnosis and prognosis may change over time. His treatment may leave him feeling fine one day and terrible the next. His emotional reserves may go from depleted to replenished then back to depleted again.
- While I (Alan) am a few years out from my diagnosis, I certainly know that at times I still ride an emotional rollercoaster, particularly when I am scheduled to return for my ongoing check-ups.
- In ever-changing circumstances like these, mood swings are normal and understandable.
- Still, no matter how normal mood swings might be for people with cancer, they don't feel good—for her or for you. It's stressful to feel yanked around like that.
- If your friend is suffering from mood swings, help her find ways to cope, such as meditation and physical activity. Planning possible ways to respond to her next mood shift may help her feel a little more prepared, a little more in control of her out-of-control life.

CARPE DIEM

Brainstorm with your friend a list of things he can try the next time he's feeling yanked around by cancer.

28.

TAKE CARE OF YOURSELF

"Rest and self-care are so important. When you take time to replenish your spirit, it allows you to serve others from the overflow. You cannot serve from an empty vessel."

— Eleanor Brown

- Being a good companion on the cancer journey is stressful. It will affect you physically, emotionally, socially, cognitively, and spiritually. To counterbalance this stress, you must make sure to take extra-good care of yourself in all five areas.

- Get enough sleep, eat healthfully, drink lots of water, and continue exercising. Your body might respond to the stress by being more susceptible to viruses, for example, but if you take good care of yourself, you're more likely to stay healthy.

- Whenever you empathize with someone who is experiencing loss, you, too, experience loss. That means you need to find ways to express your own grief. Find someone to talk to about the many thoughts and feelings you've been having.

- Socially, you need to make time for fun and enjoyable outlets and relationships. You can only be a good cancer companion in doses. In between doses you need recovery time.

- You may find that you're not thinking clearly because of the stress of helping someone through cancer. If you're experiencing cognitive challenges, that's a sign that you need to take a break from caregiving. You probably need more rest, and you may need to get others involved in helping companion the person with cancer.

- The most profound questions of cancer are spiritual questions. You will probably struggle with your religious and spiritual beliefs as you companion your friend. Be sure to make time every day to express your spirituality in whatever ways you find meaningful.

CARPE DIEM

Make a checklist of ways you will commit to taking care of yourself in all five areas as you companion this person through cancer.

29.

LIVE YOUR OWN LIFE FULLY
AND ON PURPOSE

"Grief is forever. It doesn't go away; it becomes a part of you, step for step, breath for breath. I will never stop grieving Bailey because I will never stop loving her. That's just how it is. Grief and love are conjoined; you don't get one without the other. All I can do is love her, and love the world, emulate her by living with daring and spirit and joy."

— Jandy Nelson

- Your friend's life may have been placed in jeopardy. It's devastating, and it's unfair. But consider this experience a wake-up call for your own life.

- You are alive, and we hope you are perfectly healthy. If so, you have what your friend wishes and dreams she could have. You can choose to take your good health as a sign that you still have joys to revel in, work to do, and gifts to share here on Earth.

- Many cancer patients we have talked to have told us that what they want most for their friends and family is for them to live their own lives with the understanding that every moment is truly precious. So, choose to really live. Choose to be your best self. Choose to share your unique talents. Choose to love and connect.

- Your friend's time on Earth may be diminished or cut short. Don't make his illness even more of a waste by frittering away your precious remaining years. Instead, live for yourself *and* for your friend. Make him proud of how you spend each and every day.

CARPE DIEM
Do something today that your friend would be delighted about.

30.

COMMUNE WITH NATURE

"Nature is my medicine."
— Sara Moss-Wolfe

- During times of grief and loss, many people find it restorative and energizing to spend time in nature. Returning to the natural world encourages you to discover what is essential both within you and the world around you.

- As a human being, you are a part of the natural world, and you are interdependent with it. As many naturalists would remind you, a close relationship with nature grounds your psyche and soul in the spiritual certainty of your roots. If you lose touch with nature's rhythms, you lose touch with your deepest self, with what some would call "the ground of your being."

- If you allow yourself to befriend nature, you will discover that its timeless beauty is renewing and healing. Observe how children respect and honor the spirit of nature and its beauty because they understand it instinctively. Flowers, birds, bugs, and butterflies often bring enthusiastic cries of recognition in children. You too can approach nature with the openness of a child. Take pleasure in the sounds, sights, and smells that fill your senses.

- Look up at the sky filled with beautiful clouds or twinkling stars. Stand barefoot in cool grass. Play in the snow. Taste sweet strawberries from the field. Feel the wind and sun on your skin. It doesn't matter if you are in a garden or a park, in the mountains or beside the ocean. Mother Nature will soothe your soul and refresh your spirit.

CARPE DIEM
Today, reflect on your relationship with the natural world. Go for a walk or hike and invite the Divine to come along. Allow nature to sustain you and bring you peace. As you do this, hold the person with cancer in your heart.

31.

HONOR AND EXPRESS YOUR OWN THOUGHTS AND FEELINGS

"Unexpressed emotions will never die. They are buried alive and will come forth later in uglier ways."

— Sigmund Freud

- When someone you care about has a life-changing or life-threatening illness, you will naturally grieve. You, too, are experiencing loss.

- Whenever you are experiencing feelings of loss, that means you need to express those feelings. Just as your friend with cancer needs to share her thoughts and feelings, you, too, need to share yours.

- While we encourage you to be honest about your own thoughts and feelings when you are talking to your friend with cancer, we also encourage you to find other outlets for your grief. Understandably, your friend will probably be consumed with her treatment and her own grief journey. So, it's important for you to find others to talk to and other ways to take your internal thoughts and feelings about the cancer and express them on the outside. You, too, must mourn.

- Grief is not a contest. Don't fall into the trap of thinking that because you're not the one with cancer—you're not the one whose health and maybe life are at risk—that your grief doesn't "matter." Of course your grief matters. You matter. Your well-being matters.

CARPE DIEM

Identify two or three people you can talk to whenever you need a listening ear or a shoulder to cry on as you companion your friend through cancer.

32.

MAKE SOMETHING WITH YOUR OWN TWO HANDS.

"Write it. Shoot it. Publish it. Crochet it, sauté it, whatever. MAKE."
— Joss Whedon

- The act of making something yourself is an act of creation. Creation is the opposite of destruction, which is what cancer and cancer treatment often feels like. Plus, sharing your creation with your friend with cancer is like giving him a part of yourself.

- Making art is a wonderful way to shape your thoughts and feelings into something tangible.

- Anything you make counts. Are you a baker? Bake cookies or bread. Are you a piano player? Offer to play the piano for your friend. Are you a gardener? Plant something in a pot for her so she can enjoy it year-round.

- The quality of your creation is completely beside the point. Don't worry if your efforts are thoroughly amateurish. It's the process of making and sharing that matters.

- If your friend is up to it and likes this sort of activity, offer to bring supplies to his house so he can join in on the fun.

CARPE DIEM
Make something today with your own two hands and give it to your friend.

33.

MAKE HIM A MIXTAPE

"Music is the shorthand of emotion."
— Leo Tolstoy

- We know, we know. They're not really mixtapes anymore. They're more likely to be playlists. But whatever you call them, a carefully chosen and ordered compilation of songs together on one CD or playlist might be something your friend with cancer will be glad to have. She may even want to play it over and over again throughout her cancer journey.
- Sometimes people with cancer choose a certain fight song—the song that will be their anthem as they battle cancer.
- Some songs to consider for your mixtape: "I Run for Life," by Melissa Etheridge; "Stand," by Rascal Flatts; "I Won't Back Down," by Tom Petty; "One Day You Will," by Lady Antebellum; "Take It to the Limit," by the Eagles; "Brand New Day," by Sting; "If You're Going Through Hell," by Rodney Atkins; "Faith," by George Michael; "Three Little Birds," by Bob Marley; "To Dance with Life," by Bryan Ferry; "Roar," by Katy Perry; "Anthem," by Leonard Cohen; "Jubilee," by Mary Chapin Carpenter; "Don't Carry It All," by the Decemberists; and "You Raise Me Up," by Josh Groban.
- Of course, you know your friend best, so pick songs you think will resonate with him.

CARPE DIEM
Spend an hour today making a mixtape for your friend or family member. Give it to him in a form that he can easily use.

34.

DON'T ALLOW YOUR HELP TO BE COMPROMISED BY CANCER MYTHS

"Cancer is not a death sentence, but rather a life sentence. It pushes one to live."
— Marcia Smith

• Don't let your empathy for or availability to your friend be negatively affected by common cancer myths. Here are some truths:
  - *Cancer is not contagious.* You can't catch it like you would a virus or bacteria. You don't need to be afraid of touching your friend or handling dishes. Do use good hygiene, though, because your friend may be more at risk of getting sick from germs.
  - *Cancer is not a death sentence.* Because of medical advances in detection and treatment, people are living longer with cancer. Some types and stages of cancer are becoming more chronic than life-threatening illnesses. The five-year survival rate for some cancers now exceeds 90 percent.
  - *Sugar, artificial sweeteners, cell phones, power lines, and antiperspirants do not cause cancer.* Scientific studies have disproven all of these myths (although obesity has been proven to be associated with certain cancers).
  - *You cannot cure cancer with a positive attitude alone.* While having a positive attitude may help your friend during her treatment and recovery, there is no scientific evidence linking a person's attitude to her risk of developing or dying from cancer. Be careful about suggesting that she'll be fine as long as she "thinks positive." This implies that if she doesn't do well, it's because her attitude wasn't good enough.

CARPE DIEM
If your friend wants to talk about what may have caused her cancer, be a good listener as she shares her thoughts and feelings. Refrain from passing along judgmental conjecture or myths about possible causes.

35.

ACT NORMAL

"I am not my cancer and it does not define me."
— Clarissa Tan

- Always remember that the person with cancer is, in many ways, the same person she always was. Yes, her cancer has altered her life experience, and she will change physically, emotionally, socially, cognitively, and spiritually as a result of her cancer. But even as all of this is happening, she is still her. She is not her cancer.

- How do you be a good friend to someone with cancer? The same ways in which you be a good friend to someone without cancer, really. Most of the ideas in this book apply to relationships and friendships regardless of health.

- If you're squeamish about medical matters, tell the person with cancer this. You don't have to know or see all the gory details to be there for him. But if you avoid him because he looks sick or because he has visible signs of his cancer or treatment, you're letting the relatively unimportant physical world get in the way of emotional and spiritual connection. Get over it. Teach yourself to see past the body to the soul beneath.

- If you're someone who usually runs from emotionally heavy circumstances and conversations, find the courage inside yourself to stick this one out. If the person with cancer is someone important to you, she needs and deserves your unconditional support in the coming months.

- Act normal. Don't pretend nothing is going on, but don't assume cancer is the only thing she wants to think or talk about, either. Be yourself. Allow the person with cancer to be herself, even as her life story is evolving.

CARPE DIEM
What's the most normal way you'd reach out to this person—the way you would have done before his diagnosis? Today, do that.

36.

HELP HER WORK ON
HER BUCKET LIST

"The bitterest tears shed over graves are for words left unsaid and for deeds left undone."
— Harriet Beecher Stowe

- People with cancer often feel a sense of panic about all the things they haven't finished and all the bucket-list items still not crossed off. At the same time, they typically begin to understand which of the things really "matter" and which are no longer important to them.

- No matter what your friend's prognosis is, she may express regret over unfinished business or a sense of urgency about wanting to finish certain things *right now*. This is a normal reaction to an abnormal situation. You can ease her mind and heart by offering to help.

- Some of the things on your friend's to-do list may be impossible to complete, but others probably aren't. Start with the ones that feel most urgent or disquieting to him. Be practical and resourceful. Reach out to other friends and family to marshal resources. If you're not good at project management, ask someone else to act as project manager while you play lackey.

- Keep in mind that the to-do list will change over the coming weeks and months, so don't think that once you've helped her take care of the items that were most urgent initially, you're done. Instead, check in with her every week or month and find out what's risen to the top, then offer to help with that. Sometimes it takes a village to help a friend with cancer.

CARPE DIEM
Work on your own unfinished-business list today.

37.

LEAVE HIM ALONE

"I hold this to be the highest task for a bond between two people—that each protects the solitude of the other."

— Rainer Maria Rilke

- People who are struggling emotionally and spiritually—and, on top of that, physically—sometimes just need to be alone. Grief and coming to terms with mortality are interior and spiritual struggles.

- Your friend's grief will naturally make her turn inward sometimes. She will naturally be depressed, and the fatigue caused by her disease and treatment as well as the normal lethargy of grief will combine to lay her low now and then. Try to understand the necessity of her stillness and solitude at these times.

- We know you would take away your friend's cancer if you could. You would also banish her emotional and spiritual pain. But you can't. No one can. And so she and she alone will need to wrestle with the thoughts and feelings inside her sometimes.

- Perhaps the trickiest part about being a cancer companion is knowing when to intrude and when to stay away. While you do need to respect boundaries and overt requests to be left alone, remember this mantra: When in doubt, reach out.

- If your friend has withdrawn, consider reaching out unobtrusively. Today's communication technologies have their downsides, but they're great for staying in touch without being a bother. You can text and e-mail often. You can write posts on his Facebook.

- You can also extend practical help without asking. Everyone has to eat. Dropping off a home-cooked meal, a few groceries, or cleaned and ready-to-eat garden vegetables is almost always a good idea.

- And do be on the watch for clinical depression (see Idea 80).

CARPE DIEM

Today, reach out to your friend who has cancer in an unexpected way. Maybe…have flowers delivered or place a bouquet on his doorstep, ring the bell, and run away!

38.

CHECK IN

"True friendship isn't about only being there when it's convenient. It's about being there when it's not."

— Author Unknown

- If the person who has cancer isn't someone you see every day, it can be hard to keep up with what's happening and make sure you stay in touch.

- Don't allow him to fall off your radar screen. Instead, make a commitment with yourself to touch base with the person at least once a week—more if appropriate.

- Set an appointment to call or visit the person. Mark it on your paper calendar or set an alarm on your phone.

- When you call or visit, make it clear that you have no expectations. It's OK if the person isn't feeling well enough to talk to you or see you. You're simply reaching out and expecting nothing in return. You'll try again next week.

- People with cancer are often abandoned by their friends and non-immediate family over time. Sometimes close family members—even those who live in the same house—can leave them feeling abandoned or forgotten. But you can be one of the few who never stops checking in.

CARPE DIEM
Right now, set a reminder to check in with your friend on a regular basis.

39.

DON'T EXPECT YOUR FRIEND TO THINK, FEEL, OR ACT IN A CERTAIN WAY

"My happiness grows in proportion to my acceptance, and in inverse proportion to my expectations."
— Michael J. Fox

• Your friend's cancer grief journey will be shaped by many factors, including:
  - his treatment regimen and prognosis
  - his life circumstances
  - his unique personality
  - his cultural and religious/spiritual background
  - his (or her!) gender
  - his support systems

• Because of these and other factors, no cancer journey is exactly the same as any other.

• Don't have rigid expectations for your friend's thoughts, feelings, and behaviors. Instead, think of your role as someone who "walks with," not behind or in front of, your friend. All along the way, invite your friend to teach you what she is thinking and feeling, and unless she is hurting herself or someone else, accept her behaviors without judgment.

CARPE DIEM
The next time you're with or talking to your friend, remember to use the "teach me" principle of learning about his cancer journey.

40.

IF YOU SCREW UP, TRY, TRY AGAIN

"Isn't it nice to think that tomorrow is a new day with no mistakes in it yet?"

— L.M. Montgomery

- Being a good friend to someone with cancer can be tricky. Depending on lots of circumstances, including your friend's personality, the other friends and family in her life, your pre-existing relationship with her, the course of the cancer, and many other variables, what she may find helpful and what she may find offensive or annoying at any given moment can be hard to predict.

- So, if you make a mistake or you end up doing or saying something that upsets him in some way, try not to take it too personally. This is your friend's cancer journey, after all, and you are there to support him. If you accidentally step on toes, simply offer a heartfelt apology and try again.

- Keep in mind the literal definition of the word "compassion": with passion. Caring for your friend "with passion" can mean with love but also with tenacity and appropriate assertiveness. Don't make a nuisance of yourself, but don't quit trying, either.

- The most common lament we hear from people who've traveled the cancer journey is that their friends and even family members abandon them over time. Don't be one of those people. Keep going back.

CARPE DIEM

Do you owe your friend with cancer (or someone else) an apology? If so, apologize in person (or over the phone, if you're far away) today.

41.

RESPECT CONFIDENTIALITY

"With a secret like that, at some point the secret itself becomes irrelevant. The fact that you kept it does not."
— Sara Gruen

- What's happening with our bodies feels very private to most of us. We might share physical news and stories with certain close friends and family members but not with everyone.

- Your friend with cancer probably feels the same way. What she might tell you in confidence and over time is not what she would tell just anyone. With certain people it takes a long time to build trust—but just a moment to lose it. I (Alan) know that there were several people I didn't feel comfortable sharing my "cancer news" with.

- Don't assume that others are in the know about your friend's cancer. Sometimes people with cancer intentionally withhold information from employers or children, for example, and it's not your place to disregard this decision.

- So be judicious in sharing your friend's cancer news and updates. When in doubt, ask him if it's OK.

- Keep in mind that you can round up help for your friend from others without sharing too many details.

CARPE DIEM

If it's appropriate, have a talk with your friend today about how she feels about the privacy of her cancer journey.

42.

TAKE IT ONE STEP FURTHER

"Do more than is required. What is the distance between someone who achieves their goals consistently and those who spend their lives merely following? The extra mile."

— Gary Ryan Blair

- When you have a little spare time or energy, push yourself to be the best cancer companion you can be.
- Whatever your impulse is, take it one step further. For example, if you find yourself thinking about your friend, take it one step further and send her a text or give her a call. If you bought your friend a card, take it one step further by writing your favorite memory of her inside the card before mailing it.
- If you see something that reminds you of your friend, take that as a sign that you're supposed to visit him in person.
- If you watch a movie you know your friend would like, take it one step further by sending her a DVD of the movie, bringing the movie to her house and watching it with her, or getting her a Netflix subscription along with a list of movies and shows you think she'd enjoy.
- Once you get started, the habit of taking it one step further might come easily to you, and we think you'll find it mutually rewarding.

CARPE DIEM
What were you planning to do next to help your friend? How can you take it one step further?

43.

GET FAMILIAR WITH ONLINE RESOURCES

"Information can bring you choices, and choices can bring power. Educate yourself about options and choices. Never remain in the dark of ignorance."

— Joy Page

- There's a lot of cancer information on the web—so much, in fact, that it's easy to get overwhelmed. But if you're trying to learn more about your friend's cancer and treatment, it's all there, at your fingertips, free of charge, 24/7.

- The American Cancer Society's website, www.cancer.org, offers extensive, trustworthy cancer information to both those with cancer and those who care about them.

- The Association of Cancer Online Resources, or www.acor.org, is a clearinghouse for different cancer communities. If you join their multiple myeloma group, for example, you'll be welcomed into a group of nearly 2,000 people affected by that type of cancer—all of whom share ideas, answer one another's questions, and generally support each other. Similar sites include www.cancercompass.com, www.cancerforums.net, and the Discussion Boards that are part of www.cancer.org.

- Information-sharing sites such as www.caringbridge.org, www.lotsahelpinghands.com, and www.carepages.com can be a great way to keep a large or far-flung group of family and friends up-to-date on your friend's treatment and health. This might ease a lot of the pressure she's feeling to keep in touch with many different people. You can start a page for your friend on one of those sites (but ask her permission first).

CARPE DIEM

Today, check out at least one of the online cancer communities mentioned in the third bullet, above. See if you might benefit from some online support and supporting.

44.

IF YOU FEEL HELPLESS, TALK ABOUT IT...THEN TAKE ACTION

"Grief is perhaps an unknown territory for you. You might feel both helpless and hopeless without a sense of a 'map' for the journey. Confusion is the hallmark of a transition. To rebuild both your inner and outer world is a major project."

— Ann Grant

• It's not uncommon for friends and family members to feel helpless, weak, or demoralized in the wake of a chronic illness like cancer. After all, you're helpless to take away your friend's cancer. You're helpless to prevent his suffering. If you feel helpless, talk about your feelings of helplessness with someone who's a good listener.

• But you have many resources within yourself. Although you are helpless to control the disease, you are far from helpless.

• Here are some ways to take action:
  - Implement the ideas in this book.
  - Focus on at least one small thing you can do each day or each week to help your friend.
  - Inform yourself about the disease.
  - Talk with other people facing similar problems.
  - Get involved in exchanging information, reaching out to others, or supporting research.
  - Discuss your feelings with a friend, doctor, social worker, psychologist, or clergyperson.

CARPE DIEM
Today, tell someone about your feelings of helplessness then take one small, helpful action.

45.

IF YOU FEEL GUILTY, TALK TO SOMEONE ABOUT IT

"Mistakes are part of life. Everyone makes them. Everyone regrets them. But, some learn from them. It's up to you to decide if you'll use your mistakes to your advantage."

— Meredith Sapp

- It's common for friends and family members of someone who has cancer to feel guilty about their own relative good health. If you're older than the person with cancer or if you have grown children and his are still young, you might think, "Why wasn't it me?" If the person with cancer has taken good care of himself and you have not, you might think, "He doesn't deserve that…but I do!"

- Alternately, it's not unusual to feel secretly relieved. "Thank goodness it's not me/my children/my husband, etc.," we might think. This sense of relief can then create what we call "relief-guilt," in which you feel relieved but also guilty about feeling relieved.

- While not everyone feels these feelings, rest assured that it's normal if you do. Feeling relieved does not make you a bad person any more than feeling guilty makes you virtuous. Life-threatening illness simply stirs up a stew of really complex thoughts and feelings. Human beings are the only species we know of that lives with an awareness of its own mortality. And being human means coming to terms with dying when we are alive—a task that is never easy.

- If you feel guilty about your friend's cancer, talk to someone about it. Expressing your own thoughts and feelings about his cancer journey is an essential part of *your* journey.

- Be careful, though, about sharing your guilty feelings with the person who has cancer. It's important for you to be open and honest, but it's also important not to overburden her with your own grief.

CARPE DIEM

If you're feeling any form of guilt or regret about your friend's cancer, talk to someone about it today.

46.

IF YOU FEEL SCARED, TALK TO SOMEONE ABOUT IT

"Fear makes us feel our humanity."
— Benjamin Disraeli

- Fear is a normal part of being a cancer companion. When it comes right down to it, death and dying are scary. And even if your friend is nowhere near death and may live for decades more, even the idea of her having a life-threatening illness (that may recur in the future) can be terrifying.

- Find ways to learn more about what you're afraid of. You can write a "fear inventory" in your journal, for example. Make a list of everything that scares you about your friend's cancer. In writing everything down, you might come to understand more about your fears and yourself.

- Sometimes you can *do something* about some of your fears, and as Joan Baez famously said, taking action is always a good antidote to despair. For example, if you're afraid that your friend could get very sick and die without realizing how important he is to others, you could plan a gathering of friends and family *now*, or you could send a request to everyone asking that they write your friend long letters telling him what he means to them. If you're afraid that you or someone else you love might also have cancer, schedule check-ups.

- Try to not be afraid of your fear. It is your friend because it is giving you valuable information: What you are most afraid of tells you what is most important to you. And identifying what is most important to you can help you live each and every precious day you have left on this Earth to the fullest.

CARPE DIEM
Finish this sentence: "I'm just so afraid that
_____." Now share this thought with
someone else, and, if appropriate, make a plan to do something
about it.

47.

IF YOU FEEL ANGRY, TALK TO SOMEONE ABOUT IT

"Bitterness is like cancer. It eats upon the host. But anger is like fire. It burns it all clean."

— Maya Angelou

- Anger is a common and understandable response after a friend's cancer diagnosis.

- *It's not fair!* we think. *He's too young!* or *She's taken good care of herself!* or *He has too many people counting on him!*

- After a cancer diagnosis and throughout the course of treatment, sometimes our anger gets directed at a certain person, such as a doctor, or at an entity, such as an insurance company. We can also feel angry with others for what we perceive they did or did not do that may have contributed to our friend's illness.

- Anger, rage, and blame are, at bottom, protest emotions. They are how we protest a reality that we wish were not true. As with all feelings in grief, anger is neither good nor bad, right nor wrong. It simply is. And it needs to be expressed in order to be worked through.

- With anger, it's important that its expression does not physically or emotionally hurt someone else (or even ourselves). Find more neutral ways to express anger, such as intense physical activity or talking with a friend or counselor.

CARPE DIEM

Are you angry about your friend's cancer? If you are, share your angry thoughts and feelings with a neutral but compassionate friend today.

48.

GIVE TO THE CAUSE

"Happiness exists on earth, and it is won through prudent exercise of reason, knowledge of the harmony of the universe, and constant practice of generosity."

— José Martí

- Financial giving is not only a way of supporting a cause: it's a way to affirm to yourself what you believe is important.
- "Putting your money where your mouth is" is a kind of ritual, really. It's a physical act that gives concrete, practical shape to your passions and values.
- There's probably a nonprofit working to prevent or cure the specific type of cancer your loved one has. The American Cancer Society and other general cancer nonprofits also do amazing work. Consider supporting them with a financial gift in your friend's name. Alternately, you might choose to support a different, non-cancer-related cause that is near and dear to your friend's heart.
- How much you are able to give is less important than the act of giving. Every dollar makes a difference.

CARPE DIEM
Mail a check or make an online donation today.

49.

BECOME A BONE MARROW DONOR

"It was a moment I will savor for the rest of my life. Just knowing my life was so valuable to someone else was almost incomprehensible."

— Alec, on the moment he found out he was a bone marrow "match"

- Cancer patients whose next step (and maybe last chance) is a bone marrow or blood stem cell transplant are so grateful for donors. About 30 percent of these patients will find a match within their own families, but the remaining 70 percent must rely on finding a match from the worldwide database of volunteer donors.

- Leukemias and lymphomas (blood cancers) are often treated with bone marrow or cord blood transplants. Patients with other types of cancer may also be candidates.

- The first step in becoming a possible donor is learning more about the process. Visit www.bethematch.org, which is operated by the National Marrow Donor Program, for more information.

- About one in 500 people who signs up for the registry will end up being a match for a transplant. You do not actually donate marrow unless and until you are a match.

- If you can't be a bone marrow donor, perhaps you can donate blood and/or opt in as an organ donor.

CARPE DIEM
Look into becoming a bone marrow or blood stem cell donor today.

50.

LIVE IN THE NOW

"What day is it?"
"It's today," squeaked Piglet.
"My favorite day," said Pooh.

— A.A. Milne

- You may have heard it said that there is no past, there is no future, there is only this moment.

- In his bestselling book *The Power of Now*, Eckhart Tolle encourages us to truly be present in the current moment. "Life is now," he writes. "There was never a time when your life was not now, nor will there ever be… Nothing ever happened in the past; it happened in the Now. Nothing will ever happen in the future; it will happen in the Now."

- The challenge is that it is really *hard* to live in the moment. Our minds constantly revisit the past and think forward to the future. Our egos dwell on what was and what will be. Especially when we are uncertain about our futures, we tend to obsess about what *could* happen. Uncertainty makes us anxious.

- The next time you find yourself ruminating about what *might* happen, consciously pull yourself to the present moment. Look— really look—at your surroundings. Take a deep breath and discern what you smell. Reach out to touch several different textures within arm's reach. Listen to the sounds you hear. Consider the power of Now and revel in this moment.

CARPE DIEM

Right now, empty your mind of its concerns and just "be" in this moment. Breathe in; breathe out. Find at least one thing around you to marvel about or give thanks for. Model living in the Now for your friend.

51.

PACK A CHEMO CARE KIT

"During chemo, you're more tired than you've ever been. But you also find that you're stronger than you've ever been. You're clear. Your mortality is at optimal distance, not so up close that it obscures everything else, but close enough to give you depth perception."

— Melissa Bank

- People who undergo chemotherapy often suffer in many ways. You can help make their experience a little more tolerable by helping pack (and restocking, when it runs low) a chemo care kit in an attractive tote bag.

- Chemo causes dry mouth and oral discomfort. Pack her favorite hard candy and mouthwash. Canker sores are common, so a mouth gel such as Zilactin-B can be helpful.

- Nausea is a famously awful chemo side effect. Look for ginger gum and hard candies, because anything gingery helps soothe nausea. Vomit bags also come in handy. "Borrow" a few on your next airplane flight or buy some at your local drugstore.

- Chemo can cause nerve damage in the feet, so cushy socks with treads on the bottom might be safer for your friend to wear around the house than regular socks. A travel blanket and neck pillow will help him stay warm and maybe even get some rest as he sits in the chemo chair.

- Sanitizing hand wipes will help protect your friend's compromised immune system.

- Don't forget to include some fun items to help pass the time—a book of crossword puzzles, a page-turner novel, magazines, a simple handheld electronic game (such as Sudoku).

CARPE DIEM

If your friend is or will be undergoing chemo, pack a care kit today. Your neighborhood pharmacist may have some suggestions if you're not sure what to include.

52.

FOSTER HOPE

"Once you choose hope, anything's possible."
— Christopher Reeve

- Hope is an expectation of a good that is yet to be. No matter what your friend's prognosis is, he can have hope for good things—big or small—that may yet happen.

- Hope is a bit different from optimism, which is a general feeling that good things will happen. Both are beneficial, but hope comes from having goals and dreams together with the desire and plans to reach them.

- Fostering hope in a friend with cancer is different than thumbing your nose at a grim prognosis. When you say things like, "Of course you're going to pull through this" or "I just know a miracle is coming," you're not helping anyone—your friend, her family, yourself—acknowledge and embrace the reality of what may come. It's like sending a card that says "Get Well" to a Stage-IV cancer patient. She's almost certainly not going to get well. She may live for much longer than anyone expected, but she will battle the disease for the rest of her life.

- Instead, fostering hope means helping your friend have things to look forward to. Yes, for cancer patients with certain types and stages of cancer, this often means getting through treatment and living cancer-free. But for many others with cancer, fostering hope will mean having outings and get-togethers on the calendar, achieving small goals, taking care of unfinished business, and reveling in the joy and beauty each day brings. Regardless of prognosis, you can help nurture hope in these ways.

CARPE DIEM
Today, find one small way to help build hope into your friend's life.

53.

EXPRESS YOUR SPIRITUALITY...

"Above all, cancer is a spiritual practice that teaches me about faith and resilience."

— Kris Carr

• Above all, grief is a spiritual journey of the heart and soul. Illness and loss invite you to consider why people live, why people die, and what gives life meaning and purpose. These are the most spiritual questions we have language to form.

• You can discover spiritual understanding in many ways and through many practices—prayer, worship, and meditation among them. You can nurture your spirituality in many places—nature, church, temple, mosque, monastery, retreat center, or kitchen table. No one can "give" you spirituality from the outside in. Even when you gain spiritual understanding from a specific faith tradition, the understanding is yours alone, discovered through self-examination, reflection, and spiritual transformation.

• Mourning invites you down a spiritual path at once similar to that of others yet simultaneously your own. The reality that you have picked up this book shows that you are seeking to understand and embrace your cancer grief as you help a friend embrace hers. Sometimes this happens within a faith tradition through its scriptures, community of believers, and teachers. Other times a book is just what you need to support and gently guide you in ways that bring comfort and hope.

CARPE DIEM

If you attend a place of worship, visit it today, either for services or an informal time of prayer and solitude. If you don't have a place of worship, perhaps you have a friend who seems spiritually grounded. Ask her how she learned to nurture her spirituality. Sometimes, someone else's ideas and practices provide just what you need to stimulate your own spiritual self-care.

54.

...BUT DON'T PROSELYTIZE
ABOUT YOUR OWN RELIGION

"I love you when you bow in your mosque, kneel in your temple, pray in your church. For you and I are sons of one religion, and it is the spirit."

— Kahlil Gibran

• Your faith may be so strong that you're sure there's life after death and that your friend will be happy and loved for eternity. Still, now is not the time for missionary work. Unless your friend asks, try to keep your beliefs to yourself.

• A more appropriate idea is to invite your friend to your church or place of worship with you, particularly if she doesn't attend one of her own. If she declines, don't push.

• Remember that having faith and mourning aren't mutually exclusive. A person can be very faithful yet still mourn the many losses he is experiencing.

• Now *is* the time, on the other hand, to let your friend teach you about her beliefs or listen to her as she expresses aloud her questions and pain over issues of faith. Witness and honor her unique journey.

CARPE DIEM
If your beliefs are different than your friend's and you are struggling with this, be sure to talk to someone else about your turmoil.

55.

MAKE TIME FOR MEMORIES

"Nothing is ever really lost to us as long as we remember it."
— L.M. Montgomery

• As we've said, one important need of mourning is to remember. As your friend moves through her cancer journey, your thoughts will at times naturally turn to your memories of her. This is normal and necessary. Your friend, too, will need to remember and reminisce.

• When either of you has these urges and moments of remembering, take the time to slow down and really explore them. Share them with each other. Look through old photos and watch old videos. Retell old stories.

• Your friend may appreciate the gift of sorting through and organizing his photos, whether in photo albums or on his computer. This is also an activity you can do together or you can do while he rests.

• If your loved one will be spending a lot of time in the hospital or in her bed, you can help by making sure she has photos handy. Buy a photo collage frame and fill it with special photos, then bring it to her hospital room or hang it on her bedroom wall. Or put together a slide show that can run on her laptop.

• A number of online companies such as www.collage.com offer products such as photo quilts and blankets that make lovely, useful gifts for someone who is ill. Simply upload a batch of photos and their easy-to-use design system does the rest.

CARPE DIEM
Get out some old photos today and spend at least half an hour reminiscing.

56.

PRAY

---

*"On the day I called, you answered me; my strength of soul
you increased."*

— Psalms 138:3

- While not everyone is a believer in prayer or feels helped by it, most
  of the people with cancer whom we have known welcomed prayers
  on their behalf. And for people who do pray, prayer is a time of
  meditation, contemplation, and hope.

- Prayer is not only an attempt to connect with a higher power. It
  is also mourning, because prayer involves taking your feelings and
  articulating them to someone else. Even when you pray silently,
  you're forming words for your thoughts and feelings and you're
  offering up those words to a presence outside yourself.

- If you believe in a higher power, pray. Pray for your friend. Pray for
  others affected by his cancer. Pray for your own health. Pray for your
  questions about life and death to be answered. Pray for the strength
  to persevere as a cancer companion and to find continued meaning
  in life and living.

- Many places of worship have prayer lists. Call yours and ask that
  your friend's name be added to the prayer list. On worship days, the
  whole congregation will pray for her. Often many individuals will
  pray at home for those on the prayer list, as well.

CARPE DIEM
Bow your head right now and say a silent prayer. If you are out of
practice, don't worry; just let your thoughts flow naturally.

57.

REACH OUT AND TOUCH

"Sometimes, reaching out and taking someone's hand is the beginning of a journey."

— Vera Nazarian

- For most of us, physical contact with other human beings is healing. Touch has been recognized since ancient times as having transformative, healing powers. Touch is also a way of connecting, literally and spiritually, with someone you care about.

- Your friend with cancer may or may not be someone you would usually hug, but under these circumstances, we urge you to integrate touch into your relationship. We have found that when they are sick and vulnerable, people's defenses naturally come down, and even non-huggers often start accepting, even craving, hugs and other forms of touch.

- If you sense that your touch would we welcomed, you can make hugs part of your ritual with this person. Hug him whenever you see him, then hug him again before you leave. Also consider other subtle but powerful ways you can offer touch whenever you are together, such as holding hands, rubbing his neck and shoulders, tucking a blanket around him, assisting him with grooming, and giving him a foot massage or manicure.

- As you grieve your friend's cancer, it's important for you, too, to be touched. Hug someone you feel safe with. Get a full-body massage. Kiss your children or a friend's baby. Walk arm in arm with a neighbor.

CARPE DIEM
Try hugging your close friends and family members today, even if you usually don't. You just might like it!

58.

FIND ACTIVITIES TO DO TOGETHER

"A day spent with friends is a day well spent."
— Author Unknown

- One way of being present to someone is to really listen to them as they talk. But even engaged, meaningful conversation grows fatiguing after a while, and for cancer patients who aren't feeling well or are tired of talking about their problems, heart-to-hearts can get tiresome. For those times, have activities at the ready.

- Some people really enjoy playing cards or board games, but in the busyness of regular life, rarely get a chance. Now may be the perfect time to rekindle that pastime. Scrabble, backgammon, and chess are old standbys. And your local game or bookstore stocks lots of fantastic newer options.

- Some people, especially when they are in the hospital or bedridden at home, love the simple pleasure of being read aloud to. Bring a novel or nonfiction book in a genre he likes, or offer to read the newspaper or a magazine.

- For up-and-around days, the two of you can go for a walk (outdoors or in the mall), out to lunch, fishing, for a drive, or on a day trip somewhere interesting. Or take a one-time class together (think cooking, meditation, or photography).

CARPE DIEM
Today, make a list of at least 10 things you could do together with your friend who has cancer. Now plan on doing one of them with him this week.

59.

OFFER COGNITIVE COPING TIPS AND FUN

"When you hear the word 'cancer,' it's as if someone took the game of Life and tossed it into the air. All the pieces go flying. Everything has shifted. You don't know where to start."

— Regina Brett

- Although the correlation isn't well understood, chemotherapy seems to cause thinking and memory problems for many people. Your friend might seem to be spacey or not thinking clearly. This is a common challenge for cancer patients—so common that there are names for it. You might hear your friend call these times of chemotherapy-related cognitive impairment or dysfunction "chemo brain" or "chemo fog."

- If your friend is frustrated by chemo brain, help him find ways to adapt. For example, he may need to write things down in a notebook he always keeps by his side or take care of cognitively challenging tasks early in the day, when he seems to think better.

- Memory and thinking games can help repair your friend's broken brain circuits. Offer to play Scrabble, chess, Bananagrams, or Boggle with her.

- Bring brainy gifts, like crossword puzzles and books. Read a book to or with her then discuss it.

- A number of websites offer free, fun brain-training games for adults. Try www.mindgames.com or www.sharpbrains.com. Or visit www.aarp.org and search "brain games."

CARPE DIEM
If you think she would like it, consider sending your friend a brain game today. Better yet, sit down and play it with her.

60.

SCHEDULE SOMETHING THAT GIVES YOU PLEASURE EACH AND EVERY DAY

"I'm dying and I'm having fun. And I'm going to keep having fun every day I have left. Because there's no other way to play."

— Randy Pausch

- When someone we're close to is in the middle of cancer treatment or struggling with a bleak prognosis, life can be hard.

- Part of my own (Alan) early experience with cancer was *anhedonia,* which is a clinical term that therapists sometimes use to describe the flatness of depression. *An* means "without" and *hedonia* means "pleasure." I know my closest friends and family were affected by my anhedonia, which made it harder for them to be happy as well.

- To counterbalance the natural difficulties of being a cancer companion, and to fight anhedonia, purposefully plan something you enjoy doing into every day.

- Reading, baking, going for a walk, having lunch with a friend, playing computer games—do whatever brings you enjoyment.

- You'll not only enjoy life more, but you'll be a better cancer companion if, without fail, you intentionally seek pleasure each and every day.

CARPE DIEM
Right now, think of something you can do today that you enjoy.

61.

BE HIS JESTER

"Yes, they're fake. The real ones tried to kill me."
— Author Unknown

- Over and over, people with cancer have told us that one of the things they often need is a good laugh.
- You've probably heard the story of Norman Cousins, who claimed to have cured himself of a serious illness by watching funny movies. More recently, studies have proven that laughter helps lessen pain, lower stress-related hormones, and boost the immune system, among other benefits.
- Laughter also restores hope and assists us in surviving the pain of grief. If you're of faith, perhaps you'll relate to Proverbs 15:13: "A merry heart is good medicine for the soul."
- No matter your friend's diagnosis or prognosis, it's OK for both of you to laugh. In fact, it's essential to laugh! Laughter will make her body and her spirit feel better.
- If you're a naturally funny person, keep up the jokes and funny banter. Pay attention to what your friend finds funny, and supply her with her brand of comedy movies, humorous books, and links to silly videos online.

CARPE DIEM
Send your friend a funny movie or gag gift today.

62.

CRY...AND ACCEPT CRYING

*"Sometimes allowing yourself to cry is the scariest thing you'll ever do.
And the bravest. It takes a lot of courage to face the facts, stare loss in
the face, bare your heart, and let it bleed. But it is the only way to
cleanse your wounds and prepare them for healing."*

— Barbara Johnson

- When you're grieving your friend's illness, tears are a natural cleansing and healing mechanism. Crying, if you feel the urge, is normal and necessary. What's more, tears are a form of mourning. They are sacred!

- On the other hand, don't feel bad if you aren't crying a lot. Not everyone is a crier. Some men, in particular, do not feel the need to cry. The inability to cry is not necessarily a deficit.

- Your friend may also cry from time to time. If she cries in your presence, you may feel uncomfortable. As a culture, we're often not so good at witnessing others in pain.

- But it's good for your friend to cry. You can help by allowing her to cry without trying to soothe away her tears or telling her, "Don't cry..." In fact, cry along with her if you feel like crying.

- Instead of shushing your friend's tears, try reaching out and holding his hand or arm as he cries. Let him sob as long and as hard as he needs to.

CARPE DIEM
Put a travel pack of tissues in your purse or coat pocket so you'll have them handy as you companion your friend on the cancer journey.
Restock as needed.

63.

HELP TAKE CARE OF YOUR FRIEND'S FAMILY

"Family is not an important thing. It's everything."
— Michael J. Fox

- Understandably, people with cancer often worry more about their families than they worry about themselves. Especially if they have younger children, parents with cancer are anxious about what would happen if their spouses had to go it alone or, for single parents, how their kids would be cared for. People with cancer who are married or part of a long-term relationship worry about their partners.

- You can help by finding opportunities to help take care of your friend's family. Providing meals, playing chauffeur, cleaning, babysitting, offering financial assistance, and accompanying or taking them on outings are all ways you can help fill the gap.

- The great thing about helping take care of your friend's family is that you're helping everyone involved. Your friend will feel less anxious, his family will get some much-needed assistance, and you will reap the rewards of reaching out and connecting.

- If you're worried about stepping on toes, talk to your friend first about your desire and ideas for helping her family.

CARPE DIEM
Today, do something, whether big or very little, to help your friend's family.

64.

MAKE FITNESS A PRIORITY

"Movement is medicine for creating change in a person's physical, emotional, and mental states."
— Carol Welch

- If you're not fit and healthy, you won't have the energy or stamina to be the most effective cancer companion you could be. What's more, physical activity will help you cope with the stress of having a friend with cancer. Your friend also needs to stay as fit as possible throughout her treatment, because having a strong body will help her feel better as well as boost her immune system to fight the cancer.

- Yes, people who are undergoing cancer treatment need extra rest. But when possible, they also need exercise. Regular physical activity helps them maintain function, strength, and range of motion. It also lessens fatigue and nausea, improves self-esteem, and, thanks to the "happy" chemicals our bodies release when we exercise, such as endorphins, dopamine, and serotonin, raises spirits.

- You might be able to motivate your friend to get or stay fit—and take your own fitness up a couple notches at the same time. What's great is that you can spend time with your friend talking and connecting *as you exercise together.*

- Find something that both of you like to do. Walking is an option for almost everyone (and is important for cancer patients undergoing some forms of treatment, to prevent pneumonia). Some people play tennis. Others golf. Some attend classes together, such as yoga or spinning. And don't forget simple weight lifting. It preserves and builds muscle mass, which can be extremely important for people who've been weakened by chemotherapy.

- If your friend is very weak, consult with his doctor or a physical therapist about what's an appropriate starter activity.

CARPE DIEM
Get physical today. If possible, invite your friend to join you.

65.

BE A SOUNDING BOARD
AND PUNCHING BAG

"If you are upset with another's words towards you, be cautious of your reactions, for you are only meant to be a sounding board for his soul."
— Jeremy Aldana

- People with cancer have lots of thoughts and feelings inside, and they need to express those thoughts and feelings to live and love as fully as possible. In other words, they need to mourn. And as a cancer companion, you can be a receiver of their mourning.

- Sometimes people with cancer just want to run thoughts and ideas past someone else. Simply speaking those ideas out loud helps them move forward. You can listen.

- Sometimes people with cancer just need to vent (as we all do!). They get angry and frustrated and whiny, and they need to let all that anger and frustration out. You can be one of the few who will listen and empathize without judging or trying to "fix it."

- And sometimes people with cancer need a scapegoat. They feel crappy or poorly treated, and they need someone to blame. Don't be surprised if you end up being the target of their wrath or irritation one day. Try not to take it too personally. It's usually their circumstances talking—not their true beliefs.

- If you're on the receiving end of a lot of hurt and hate, don't forget to get support for yourself from someone else. You, too, will need to express your thoughts and feelings about what is being said. Attending a support group for cancer companions might be especially helpful to you if your loved one grows angry or hateful.

CARPE DIEM
If the person with cancer is especially angry or mean right now, talk to other friends and family members about how best to help him. Remember, his anger is usually a protest against underlying feelings of helplessness and fear.

66.

HELP YOUR FRIEND
WRANGLE WORRY

"If a problem is fixable, if a situation is such that you can do something about it, then there is no need to worry. If it's not fixable, then there is no help in worrying. There is no benefit in worrying whatsoever."

— Dalai Lama XIV

- Naturally, people with cancer tend to worry a lot. They worry about what will happen—if their cancer will go into remission, if it will return, how they will pay for treatment, what will happen to their families if they die—and on and on and on. The worries are endless. And understandable.

- We've said that feelings aren't right or wrong, they just are. This is true of worry too. Encouraging your friend to express his worry every time he's feeling it is the ticket. Here are some techniques for both of you to try:
    - Make a written list of your worries.
    - Look over the list and decide which worries you can do something about—and then do it.
    - If your friend is worried about who would take care of his children if he couldn't, for example, arrange a conversation between him and the person whom he would like to serve as guardian.
    - Practice living in the Now (see Idea 50).
    - Talk to several different people about your biggest worries.
    - See a grief counselor.
    - Cry, scream, punch a punching bag.

CARPE DIEM

What is your friend's biggest worry right now? Can you help her *do* something about it? If you can, take steps today to begin to put that worry to rest. If you can't, at least encourage her to talk it through.

67.

LEARN TO MEDITATE

"Cancer taught me to live only in the day I'm in. In the moment I'm in. Some moments, I simply ground myself by touching the desk, the table, the wall wherever I am and say, 'You're right here. Stay put in this moment.'"

— Regina Brett

- Meditation is simply quiet, relaxed contemplation. It's a great way to ease tension and anxiety. It's also a way to get in touch with your truest thoughts and feelings.

- You needn't follow any particular rules or techniques in order to meditate. Simply find a quiet place where you can focus without distraction and rid your mind of superficial thoughts and concerns.

- Relax your muscles and close your eyes if you'd like.

- Focus on your breath. When your mind starts thinking its monkey thoughts (which it will!), return your focus to breathing in and out.

- Try meditating for 10 to 15 minutes each day. It may help center you and provide a time of respite from your cancer grief and companioning.

- If you've tried meditating in the past and have discovered that it's not a good fit for you, that's OK. Meditation isn't for everyone. Try other techniques instead.

CARPE DIEM

If you're unsure how to get started on meditating, try listening to guided audio meditations. You can find a number of free ones online, including these on the UCLA Mindful Awareness Research Center website: www.marc.ucla.edu/body.cfm?id=22.

68.

START A CARE CALENDAR

"Never doubt that a small group of thoughtful, committed citizens can change the world. Indeed, it's the only thing that ever has."

— Margaret Mead

- No matter how willing you are to help your friend through his cancer journey, you can't do it alone. The more people who get involved in helping, the better.

- One way to plug lots of people into the routine of helping your friend and her family is by using a care calendar. They're free and available on lots of websites, including www.caringbridge.org and www.carecalendar.org.

- A care calendar is a place people can sign up to provide meals, carpool kids, do yard work, accompany the patient to chemo, and all the other things that need doing.

- Some care calendars also have room to give status updates, so helpers know what's happening with the patient's health and treatment.

- Appointing someone as keeper of the calendar will help ensure it stays up-to-date and that your friend gets all the help he needs.

CARPE DIEM
Start an online care calendar for your loved one today.

69.

BEWARE THE NOCEBO EFFECT

"Beliefs have the power to create and the power to destroy. Human beings have the awesome ability to take any experience of their lives and create a meaning that disempowers them or one that can literally save their lives."

— Anthony Robbins

- Have you heard of the nocebo effect? It's the placebo effect's evil twin.

- As you know, the placebo effect is the improvement of symptoms or outcomes based simply on belief. If a doctor gives you a sugar pill but tells you that it is medicine that will make you better, you are, in fact, more likely to get better than others who didn't receive the placebo pill.

- The nocebo effect is the opposite. People who are warned about pain or side effects before a treatment are, studies prove, more likely to report pain or side effects afterward.

- The mind is a powerful creator. Thoughts can indeed create, or at least foster, reality.

- While it's natural to be afraid and to consider the worst after a friend's cancer diagnosis or follow-up testing, keep in mind the nocebo effect. If your friend is feeling negative, allow her to express her black thoughts while at the same time finding ways to help her nurture positivity and hope.

CARPE DIEM

If dark, pessimistic thoughts seem to be consuming you or your friend, consider talking to a counselor trained in Cognitive Behavioral Therapy. (You might also see the term Cognitive Processing Therapy.) A CBT therapist can give you tools to adjust your thought patterns. Meditation can also help you clear your mind and focus instead on a positive mantra.

70.

GET INVOLVED

"Volunteers are love in motion."
— Author Unknown

- Your friend's illness has probably made you more aware of the movement to find a cure for cancer and promote early detection.

- Consider honoring your friend by getting involved in cancer activism. Many types of cancer have their own organizations (such as the Lustgarten Foundation for Pancreatic Research) and events (such as the Susan G. Komen 3-Day walks for breast cancer). Of course, reputable general organizations such as the American Cancer Society provide support, advocacy, and funding for all types of cancer.

- My (Alan's) father died from malignant melanoma (the deadliest form of skin cancer). I help sponsor an annual run/walk in my community that raises money to help combat this horrible disease. The contribution I make every year helps me remember my dad and feel like I'm helping prevent similar deaths in the future.

- Donate money if you can. Volunteer if you have time. Give in-kind gifts (such as artwork you create or furniture you no longer need) for silent auctions and fundraisers.

CARPE DIEM
Ask your friend or look online for some suggestions about upcoming events you could participate in or campaigns you could support.

71.

LISTEN TO HER STORY...AS OFTEN AS SHE FEELS THE NEED TO TELL IT

"I know now that we never get over great losses; we absorb them, and they carve us into different, often kinder, creatures. We tell the story to get them back, to capture the traces of footfalls through the snow."

— Gail Caldwell

- Acknowledging the reality of cancer is a painful, ongoing task that people who have been diagnosed accomplish in doses, over time. For them, a vital part of healing their grief is often "telling the story" over and over again. It's as if each time they tell the story, it becomes a little more comprehensible and bearable.

- Their cancer story may begin on the day they found a lump or the moment their doctor told them the biopsy results. It might begin earlier—maybe when they first grew concerned that they carried a genetic predisposition to cancer or when a friend or family member was diagnosed. Each time they receive an additional treatment, have a new imaging scan, or experience a new side effect, a chapter is added to their story.

- You can be someone who is willing to listen to the story, without judgment, as it grows and changes over time. Remember that what to the listener might seem like repetition may be to the teller a way of understanding and accepting what is happening.

CARPE DIEM

The next time your friend shares part of her cancer story with you, try to listen with rapt and complete attention.

72.

THROW A PARTY

"It's not the years in your life that count. It's the life in your years."
— Abraham Lincoln

- If and when your friend's energy returns to him, throw him a party! What *kind* of a party depends on your friend's personality, likes, and dislikes, but the point is to have a celebration that brings friends and family together to honor his ongoing life.
- When should you have the party? As soon as makes sense! Others will want to catch up with your friend and find out the latest news, so you might as well get them all together in one room.
- What does your friend love in life? Use that as your party theme, and go over-the-top with it. If he loves biking, hold a bike parade. If he's into Star Trek, make it a costume party and play Star Trek movies nonstop in the background.
- Think about what you and everyone else would miss about your friend if she were no longer here…and use those thoughts and feelings to give you ideas for the party. We're not trying to be morbid. Rather, we're trying to encourage you to see this party as the precious opportunity that it is.

CARPE DIEM
Call a mutual friend today and start making plans for your friend's party.

73.

HOLD A FUNDRAISER

"In charity there is no excess."
— Francis Bacon

- Many people with cancer need help paying for their treatment as well as their regular bills, especially if they aren't able to work while they're in treatment. According to a Duke University Medical Center study, out-of-pocket expenses averaged over seven hundred dollars a month for doctor visits, medicines, lost wages, and travel to appointments. People undergoing chemotherapy pay the most.

- Your friend may or may not tell you that she is struggling financially, so don't be afraid to ask. "Are finances challenging because of all the medical bills and lost work?" is a not-too-nosy question that may open the door to a helpful conversation.

- There are several ways you may be able to help your friend financially. One good one is to make sure she's aware of financial resources for cancer patients in her community. Call the nearest American Cancer Society office to get started on this hunt.

- Another way to help with finances is to review your friend's insurance coverage, explanation of benefits statements, and medical bills. Mistakes are common, and sometimes hospitals and healthcare providers will write off unpaid balances under certain circumstances.

- Finally, you can organize a fundraiser! How many people do you know who would pitch in to help your friend if they were only asked?

CARPE DIEM
Talk to your friend with cancer about finances today.

74.

SHAVE YOUR OWN HEAD

"We're all born bald, baby."
— Telly Savalas

- If chemotherapy is causing your friend's hair to fall out, consider shaving your own head in solidarity. It just might be the crazy, over-the-top gesture that your friend needs right now to help him feel less alone.
- Rope other friends and family members into getting their heads shaved, too. You might be surprised by how many people will feel empowered by the act.
- If you have long hair and can cut off at least ten inches, you can donate your hair to Locks of Love or other organizations that provide free or low-cost wigs to people whose own hair has been lost to disease or medical treatment.
- Or, if you're good with hair, you might be able to help your friend select and style an attractive, well-fitting wig. Consult with her insurance company first, because the wig may be covered.

CARPE DIEM
Is your friend grieving the loss of his hair? Even if he's not normally vain, don't assume that hair loss isn't bothering him. Talk to him about it today.

75.

DON'T BE AFRAID TO "BOTHER" HIM...

"A ship is always safe at the shore, but that is not what it is built for."
— Albert Einstein

- Lots of times, those of us without cancer feel like we have to walk on eggshells when we're around people with cancer. We don't know what to say, we don't know what he needs, we don't know what's going on with his treatment right now…so we don't reach out. "We didn't want to bother you" is something cancer patients hear all the time.

- Yes, you might wake up the person with cancer if you call her on the phone. And yes, you might catch her napping if you drop by her house. But reaching out is almost *always* better than not reaching out. Connecting in sensitive, respectful ways is always better than ignoring.

- People undergoing cancer treatment learn pretty quickly how to set boundaries. If he's catching forty winks, he'll probably turn his phone off. If he can't come to the door right now, he won't come to the door. Often he has someone who serves as a "gatekeeper." Even when his gatekeeper tells you that the patient is sleeping or is feeling too sick to see anyone right now, your friend will still appreciate hearing that you tried to connect with him.

- And if you *do* end up "bothering" her? Chances are, your love and your repeated attempts to be present will far outweigh any inconvenience you may cause.

CARPE DIEM
Unless it's the middle of the night, call your friend right now. If it is the middle of the night, send him a text, e-mail, or handwritten note in the mail.

76.

...BUT DON'T OVERSTAY
YOUR WELCOME, EITHER

"When the eyes say one thing, and the tongue another, a practiced man relies on the language of the first."

— Ralph Waldo Emerson

- Throughout this book, we've been encouraging you to spend time with the person with cancer. Give the present of your presence. This is the single most important rule for cancer companions.

- Never forget, however, that, especially during treatment cycles, your friend's energy will be lower than usual. On any given day, you might be prepared to hang around for an hour or two, but your friend may only have the stamina for a 15-minute visit. Longer isn't necessarily better.

- If your friend is tired, visit for a few minutes and then leave, with the promise to return in a day or two. Or better yet, visit for a few minutes then excuse yourself and go clean his kitchen while he takes a nap!

- Watch for cues that your friend needs to rest. If she's yawning, rubbing her eyes, or looking around the room as you talk, it's probably time to skedaddle. Look for opportunities to use your "emotional intelligence."

CARPE DIEM

The next time you visit your friend, spend 15 minutes visiting and 15 minutes doing something practical (cleaning out the fridge, vacuuming, folding laundry). If you establish this as a ritual, your friend may become more accepting of your hands-on help.

77.

PAY ATTENTION TO SYNCHRONICITIES

"When you stop existing and you start truly living, each moment of the day comes alive with wonder and synchronicity."
— Steve Maraboli

- Stuff happens, the saying goes.
- The philosophy embedded in that aphorism is that things happen over which you have no control, and you need to resign yourself to the fact that life often sucks.
- Sometimes life does suck. Sometimes stuff happens. Sometimes people you care about are diagnosed with cancer. But often, if you are paying attention, if you are living on purpose, stuff happens that is nothing short of miraculous.
- At night you dream of a friend you haven't seen for years, and the next day she calls you, out of the blue. You hear a song on the car radio that perfectly captures what you're feeling that moment. Your furnace breaks down and you receive an unexpected check in the mail.
- Pay attention to such coincidences. Believe that they may be telling you something—even guiding you. As the Dalai Lama said, "I am open to the guidance of synchronicity and do not let expectations hinder my path."

CARPE DIEM

The next time you experience what feels like a coincidence, write it down on your calendar or explore it in your journal. Contemplate what guidance it may be offering.

78.

SLEEP WELL

"Sleep is the golden chain that ties health and our bodies together."
— Thomas Dekker

- How is your sleep? Nothing is more essential to your health than restful and sufficient sleep. Yet as you companion someone with cancer, you may not be sleeping well. In fact, one in three people has trouble falling or staying asleep even without the added stress of cancer.

- Cancer or no cancer, most of us get less sleep than we need, and studies show that most of us would sleep an hour longer if we could.

- A normal night's sleep consists of several distinct stages and types of sleep. Stage 1 is the twilight zone between being awake and asleep. Stage 2 sleep brings larger brain waves, and we are no longer conscious of our surroundings. In Stages 3 and 4, our brains produce slower and even larger waves, referred to as delta or slow-wave sleep.

- After about 90 minutes in the four stages of quiet sleep, the brain shifts into the more active stage characterized by rapid eye movement (REM). Brain waves during REM resemble those of wakefulness, but the large muscles of the body cannot move. This is the time of vivid dreaming. During a typical night we spend about 25 percent of the time in REM sleep and may have four or five cycles of REM sleep.

- In today's busy world, we often do not leave enough time in our lives for adequate sleep, and many people start the day off tired and rundown. Especially as you help a loved one through his cancer journey, it is essential to get the sleep you need.

CARPE DIEM

If you are not sleeping well, talk to your physician about your sleep troubles. She may have excellent sleep suggestions for people experiencing stress.

79.

MOVE

"It's helpful to realize that this very body that we have, that's sitting right here right now…with its aches and its pleasures…is exactly what we need to be fully human, fully awake, fully alive."

— Pema Chodron

- We all know how important physical activity is to our physical health, but did you know that it also has a significant effect on your mood? Research shows that exercise helps lift anxiety and ease depression.
- As you companion a friend or family member who has cancer, you will almost certainly feel tired. Caregiving and feelings of grief and loss cause fatigue. Lay your body down every day for a short rest.
- Yet at the same time, forcing yourself to get moving every day will also help you feel better.
- We often tell mourners that they need to put their grief into motion by expressing it. This movement of thoughts and feelings is what creates opportunity for positive change. Similarly, moving your body creates physical and biochemical change that supports physical as well as emotional/spiritual healing.

CARPE DIEM

Get at least half an hour of physical activity today if you're up to it—more if your fitness level is high. You don't need to go to a gym! Gardening, housework, and all kinds of everyday activities count.

80.

KNOW THE SIGNS OF CLINICAL DEPRESSION

"There are wounds that never show on the body that are deeper and more hurtful than anything that bleeds."
— Laurell K. Hamilton

- According to the National Institute of Mental Health, symptoms of clinical depression include:
  - Difficulty concentrating or remembering details
  - Fatigue and decreased energy
  - Feelings of guilt, worthlessness, and/or helplessness
  - Feelings of hopelessness and/or pessimism
  - Insomnia, early-morning wakefulness, or excessive sleeping
  - Irritability, restlessness
  - Loss of interest in activities or hobbies you used to enjoy
  - Overeating or appetite loss
  - Persistent aches or pains, headaches, cramps, or digestive problems that do not ease, even with treatment
  - Persistent sad, anxious, or "empty" feelings
  - Thoughts of suicide or suicide attempts
- Trouble is, the cancer journey and normal grief often include many of these same symptoms. However, if your friend's feelings of self-worth are low, if he is having trouble functioning on a day-to-day basis, and certainly if he is considering suicide, please get him help right away. Anti-depressant medication or other forms of treatment may be necessary and extremely effective right now.

CARPE DIEM

If you think your friend may be suffering from clinical depression, talk to her about it today. Her depression likely requires its own appointment with her primary care physician or a well-trained grief counselor who can distinguish normal, depressive grief from clinical depression.

81.

RECOGNIZE THAT THE WAY DOWN MAY BE THE WAY UP

"The soul has many secrets. They are only revealed to those who want them, and are never completely forced upon us. One of the best kept secrets, and yet one hidden in plain sight, is that the way up is the way down. Or, if you prefer, the way down is the way up."

— Father Richard Rohr

- Change and transition are inevitable in life. We see them all around us, from the changing of the seasons to the growth of children to our own aging and transformation over time.

- To move up spiritually and have a clearer understanding of and deeper appreciation for our lives, we often must first experience loss or tragedy and go down. A job, a fortune, a marriage, or a reputation has to be lost; a death has to be suffered; or a disease like cancer has to be endured. I (Alan) often say that we must descend before we can transcend.

- If we deny pain or avoid risk-taking in the first place (such as forming close relationships or pursuing a career we're passionate about), it's true that we may be able to protect ourselves from falling down into our spiritual depths, but we also keep ourselves from reaching our spiritual heights.

- In a sense, those who have gone "down" are the ones who understand "up." In order to truly grasp the glorious beauty of our lives, we may first need to experience the dark beauty of our sorrow.

CARPE DIEM

If and when your friend is ready to have this conversation, welcome his thoughts about what he has learned from his cancer. Does he see life differently than he did before the diagnosis? Has his appreciation of life changed? Has he reached a higher "up" than he ever had before? What can he see from up there?

82.

PRACTICE BREATHING IN AND OUT

"Feelings come and go like clouds in a windy sky. Conscious breathing is my anchor."

— Thich Nhat Hanh

- When we are experiencing stress and grief, sometimes what we need most is just to "be." In our goal-oriented society, many of us have lost the knack for simply living.

- Try what's called *autogenic breathing*. It's a simple yet effective way to help you relax your mind, body, and spirit.

- Breathe in very deeply for four full seconds (slowly count 1, 2, 3, 4), then hold your breath for two seconds. Next, slowly release your breath to the count of four and hold for two additional seconds. Repeat.

- You can do this any place, any time. The more often you do it, the better. Try for a minimum of 10 minutes a day a couple of times each day.

- Afterward, notice if you feel calmer physically, emotionally, cognitively, and spiritually.

CARPE DIEM

Try reflecting on this thought: "As I allow myself to mourn, I create an opening in my heart. Releasing the tensions of grief, surrendering to the struggle, means freeing myself to go forward."

83.

BE MINDFUL OF ANNIVERSARIES

"Yesterday was the three-year anniversary of my diagnosis. It is weird the way I will start to get stressed when it gets close to that date, even still. Yesterday, though, I bought a bottle of champagne and celebrated still being alive."

— A posting on Cancer Survivors Network

- Throughout your friend's cancer journey, anniversaries of all kinds—of the day she found a lump, of the day of her diagnosis, of the day she finished radiation or chemotherapy, of her birthday or wedding anniversary, of the day a friend or family member died—may be difficult for her.

- These are times that you as his cancer companion may want to note and plan ahead for. Let him know you are thinking about him on days that may be significant to him.

- If you're not sure which days seem significant to her, ask. She may feel like talking about them anyway.

- Also know that some people feel like turning inward on such days. If that's how your friend feels, that's OK too. All of us need times of contemplative silence and spiritual reflection.

CARPE DIEM
Right now, mark your friend's special days on your calendar. If you're using an electronic calendar, set reminders so you won't forget.

84.

OFFER A CHANGE OF SCENERY

"I have always been delighted at the prospect of a new day, a fresh try, one more start, with perhaps a bit of magic waiting somewhere behind the morning."

— J.B. Priestley

- Sometimes people with cancer feel stuck because the disease has a way of putting life on hold. While the Earth keeps spinning and the everyday lives of those around your friend keep going as usual, her reality may have her feeling trapped in the quicksand of her illness.
- The reality is that treatment may consume his life for a while. While people with cancer never want to "become" their cancer, they can't help but be taken over by the many appointments and tests and therapies, at least for a time.
- Sometimes feelings of aimlessness or ineffectiveness also arise. Even after your friend's initial treatment course, she may find herself frustrated if she is unable to focus, to concentrate, to get anything done. In addition to possibly being affected by chemotherapy, her brain is still trying to understand and process what happened. This is normal and essentially a form of post-traumatic stress.
- Here's where you come in: You can offer a change of scenery. Take your friend somewhere he's never been, even if it's just a short walk, bike ride, or car trip away. Our brains like novelty. Going somewhere new fosters new thoughts and feelings.

CARPE DIEM

Today, suggest an outing to somewhere your friend has never been before. If she's not up for an outing, update her resting place with new throw pillows, blankets, and maybe even a fresh coat of paint!

85.

HELP SET UP OR ORGANIZE
A HOME OFFICE

"Nothing is so fatiguing as the eternal hanging of an uncompleted task."
— William James

- People with cancer who work in an office environment might not be able to go to work for a while…but if their jobs and employers are flexible enough, they might be able to continue to work part-time from home. And working might give them a much-needed distraction and self-esteem boost, not to mention paycheck.

- You might be able to help by setting up a home office for your friend if she doesn't already have one. If budgets are tight, search for a gently used desk, chair, bookshelf, and file cabinet on Craigslist. Nice furniture can be had for very little money if you're willing to spend some time looking. And your friend's employer might consider letting her take her work computer to her house for the time being if she doesn't have a personal computer that will work.

- Even if your friend doesn't work outside the home, now might be a good time to help set up a home office or desk for organizing all the bills and paperwork that will result from his medical treatment. If he already has a home office area or organizational system for such things, maybe he could use some help with filing.

- Don't forget the simple touches that "warm up" an office space, such as framed photos and a potted plant.

CARPE DIEM
Today, ask your friend or family member if she needs or could use some help organizing a home office.

86.

DON'T BE ALARMED BY "GRIEFBURSTS"

"In the first few months of my grief, nothing could distract me from the sorrow and pain. When you quit trying to avoid the breakdowns, the grief bursts, the weeping episodes, you feel better. I don't think you can force yourself to stop. People try, but it's ultimately what keeps them from healing."

— J.S. Jacobs

- Sometimes heightened periods of sadness overwhelm us when we're in grief. These moments can seem to come of out nowhere and can be frightening and painful. Both you and your friend may experience occasional griefbursts.

- Even long after your friend or family member's diagnosis and treatment, something as simple as a sound, a smell, or a phrase can bring on a "griefburst." He might hear a name, see a building, or feel a twinge that suddenly reminds him of his cancer and all he has gone through. Or, it might happen to you.

- Try not to be alarmed by griefbursts. They're normal and sometimes necessary. Simply stop and embrace them as you would any thought or feeling.

CARPE DIEM

Has your friend experienced a griefburst in your presence? If so, talk to someone else about it as a way of processing your own thoughts and feelings.

87.

CONNECT WITH ANIMALS

"Until one has loved an animal, a part of one's soul remains unawakened."

— Anatole France

- Animals are our natural companions. In times of crisis they can steady us and bathe us in unconditional love. Animals can open our souls to the beauty of our lives. Studies show that people live longer and have more fulfilled lives when they share them with an animal companion.
- Pets invite you to focus on their needs and not be so overwhelmed by your own. Taking care of an animal allows you to feel needed and loved by your pet.
- There is a special feeling of being here and now when you are with your pet. They have souls, too, and most pet owners feel this soulful connection with their four-legged friends. The unconditional love a pet shows may be just what you need during this difficult time.
- Does your friend with cancer have a companion animal? If so, be sure to greet and treat this animal as the beloved family member she is to your friend. Also, offer to walk or talk care of your friend's pet when her health doesn't allow her to. If your friend doesn't have a pet but enjoys animals, perhaps you can arrange for pets to visit her. Therapy dogs regularly visit oncology patients at many hospitals, for example.

CARPE DIEM
Today, find a way for your friend to enjoy and be soothed by the companionship of animals.

88.

PLAN A SLEEPOVER

"I have been one acquainted with the night."
— Robert Frost

- Remember how much fun you had sleeping over at a friend's house when you were a kid? Why not recapture that experience now?
- Slumber parties are chockfull of all the things your friend with cancer might need most right now—companionship, laughter, conversation.
- If your friend is deep in the throes of chemotherapy and lives alone, she might need around-the-clock help. Maybe she would welcome a temporary roommate who could act as both nurse and companion.
- If your friend is feeling well but needs a getaway, plan an overnight at a nearby bed and breakfast.

CARPE DIEM
Find out who is caring for your friend on days that she needs 24/7 help. Don't assume. Offer your presence if more hands are needed.

89.

GIVE MORE THAN YOU TAKE

"An individual has not started living until he can rise above the narrow confines of his individualistic concerns to the broader concerns of all humanity."
— Martin Luther King, Jr.

- The greatest happiness in life always comes from what you give rather than what you get. The happiest people are givers, not takers. Most of us will never be a Mother Teresa or a Gandhi, but in general the more we give, the more we find joy.

- One of the reasons that giving more than we take is such a great pathway to happiness and purpose is because we have control over what we give—but almost none over what we get. Think of it this way: Each day we have the power to give without limit. We can choose to give kindness, to serve, to love, to be generous, and to leave the world better in some way.

- By choosing to be a cancer companion, you are making the world a better place not only for your friend, but for the world in general. The more we care and look out for each other, the better the world becomes.

- We all long for connection to something larger than ourselves. There is a connection to the universe we may not fully understand. John Izzo, a psychologist, says there are two great tasks in life—"to find ourselves and to lose ourselves." We must truly know ourselves to truly give ourselves to others. Cancer caregiving can help you both find yourself and lose yourself to a greater cause.

CARPE DIEM

Ask yourself: How did I make the world a better place in some small way today? If you can't think of anything, then be sure to get in a good deed before you go to sleep.

90.

TAKE YOUR FRIEND TO "THIN PLACES"

"Sacred places are the truest definitions of the earth; they stand for the earth immediately and forever; they are its flags and shields. If you would know the earth for what it really is, learn it through its sacred places. You become one with a spirit that pervades geologic time and space."

— N. Scott Momaday

- In the Celtic tradition, "thin places" are spots where the separation between the physical world and the spiritual world seems tenuous. They are places where the veil between heaven and Earth, between the holy and the everyday, are so thin that when we are near them, we intuitively sense the timeless, boundless spiritual world.
- There is a Celtic saying that heaven and Earth are only three feet apart, but in the thin places that distance is even smaller.
- Thin places are usually outdoors, often where water and land meet or land and sky come together. You might find thin places on a riverbank, a beach, or a mountaintop.
- Is there a thin place that is special to you? Take your friend there to feed both your spirits.

CARPE DIEM

Your thin places are anywhere that fills you with awe and a sense of wonder. They are spots that refresh your spirit and make you feel closer to God. Take your friend to a thin place today and sit in contemplative silence.

91.

BRIGHTEN UP YOUR FRIEND'S ENVIRONMENT

"Don't own so much clutter that you will be relieved to see your house catch fire."
— Wendell Berry

- Could your friend's bedroom, kitchen, or living room use a little sprucing up?
- Cancer = a lot going on. It's hectic and chaotic, especially in the early days and weeks of diagnosis and treatment. Making your friend's home a serene oasis will help soothe her and unburden her already overburdened mind and soul. Studies even prove that when your environment is cluttered, you're more likely to feel distracted and irritable.
- So if his spaces are crowded with stuff, offer to help him clear the clutter. If he doesn't want to get rid of anything, that's OK. Maybe he'd consider having some of the stuff boxed up and stored in a closet for now.
- Simply clearing off and cleaning all the horizontal surfaces—floors, tabletops, countertops, mantels, etc.—will make a world of difference.
- Now add some new pops of color in your friend's favorite patterns and hues. Think inexpensive additions like picture frames, throw blankets, and wall hangings.
- Or, maybe your friend's patio, front porch, or yard could use some attention. Enlist the help of more friends and spend a day weeding, trimming, and planting colorful flowers.

CARPE DIEM

Buy your friend a new set of sumptuous, all-cotton bed sheets in her favorite color or an appropriate pattern. When you're spending a lot of time in bed, new sheets can feel like such a wonderful luxury.

92.

TAKE CARE OF YOUR OWN PREVENTIVE HEALTH

"We don't learn the importance of anything until it's snatched from our hands."

— Malala Yousafzai

- Cancer patients tell us all the time that it makes them very upset when they find out that friends and family members are skipping simple steps for early cancer detection.
- Are you due for a check-up? Health screenings are a good way to be sure your various parts and pieces are functioning normally. Ask your doctor which screenings, including cancer screenings, are right for you.
- There are specific health screenings for men and women. For example, men over 50 should consider a prostate cancer screening. Breast cancer is the second most common cause of death for women. They should have an annual breast exam, and those over 40 (or younger, in the case of family history) should consider mammography. Women should also have regular pap smears to detect early cervical cancer.
- And don't forget all the standard tests that come with regular check-ups, such as cholesterol and blood pressure checks for heart disease, blood sugar levels for diabetes, and more.
- If you haven't had a good general physical within the past year, schedule one today. Let your friend know that his experience is teaching you to take your own health more seriously.

CARPE DIEM
Are you current on your cancer screenings? Visit the American Cancer Society website at www.cancer.org and search the phrase "screening by age" to see a list of what is needed and when.

93.

HELP SIMPLIFY YOUR FRIEND'S LIFE

"When you get cancer, it's like really time to look at what your life was and is, and I decided that everything I've done so far is not as important as what I'm going to do now."
— Herbie Mann

- Many of us today are taking stock of what's really important in our lives and trying to discard what's not.
- People with cancer can be especially overwhelmed by all their tasks and commitments, since their treatment and their natural and necessary grief take so much time and energy.
- What might be overburdening your friend right now? Offer to take charge of his to-do list and help him decide which commitments he can and should give up for now.
- Sometimes just helping your friend identify which activities and annoyances to stop (or pause for the time being) will empower him to do so.

CARPE DIEM
People with cancer often feel obligated to write thank-you notes to the people who have sent flowers, food, or other gifts. Offer to write the notes for or with him.

94.

TELL YOUR FRIEND HOW IMPORTANT HE IS TO YOU

"The regret of my life is that I have not said 'I love you' often enough."
— Yoko Ono

- Sometimes people with cancer become filled with despair. Depending on their treatment side effects and prognosis, they may struggle for reasons to get their feet out of bed in the morning.
- Tell your friend how much she matters to you. And tell her why.
- Share the reasons you value your friendship. Tell him about the qualities you admire in him. Remind him how good he is at something he does well and how much he means to the other people in his life.
- Don't assume that your friend knows how you feel. Tell her.

CARPE DIEM
Buy a "thinking of you" card and enclose a note that describes the ways in which your friend matters so much to you.

95.

REMEMBER YOUR FRIEND ON HOLIDAYS

"Blessed is the season which engages the whole world in a conspiracy of love."
— Hamilton Wright Mabie

- It's common for people struggling with health challenges and grief to feel particularly sad and vulnerable on holidays.
- Reach out on these days. A simple unexpected phone call or short visit from you may mean the world to your friend.
- If your friend is alone (or if she and her partner are alone), invite her to share the holidays with you at your house. Or offer to bring the holiday to her. You can cook and decorate while she rests in the comfort of her own home.
- Remember that the gift of your time and presence is more precious than any material gift you could send.

CARPE DIEM

What's the next holiday that's approaching? Set a reminder to reach out to your friend before the day of the holiday and find a way to include him in your plans.

96.

TAKE YOUR FRIEND ON A PILGRIMAGE

"As I make my slow pilgrimage through the world, a certain sense of beautiful mystery seems to gather and glow."
— A.C. Benson

- Pilgrimage to a sacred place is common to all religions—Christianity, Judaism, Hinduism, Islam, Native American, to name a few. The literal definition of the word "pilgrimage" is a long journey or search, especially one of exalted purpose or moral significance.
- Cancer and cancer grief certainly send us on a long search—a search for meaning, reconciliation, and peace. What search do humans undertake that has a more exalted purpose?
- Going on a pilgrimage to a sacred place is a mark of respect and often invites spiritual renewal and inner harmony to those who make the journey. From the beginning days of the Christian church, pilgrims visited the graves of the Apostles and the martyrs. The great centers of Christian medieval pilgrimage were Jerusalem, Rome, the tomb of Saint James of Compostela in Spain, and the shrine of Saint Thomas Becket in Canterbury, England.
- In your friend's spiritual tradition, what sacred places do followers visit? Would he like you to take him there?

CARPE DIEM
If your friend is up for it, make plans today to go on a pilgrimage to a sacred place that connects her to her faith or spirituality.

97.

TURN TO THE POWER OF RITUALS

"We do spiritual ceremonies as human beings in order to create a safe resting place for our most complicated feelings of joy or trauma, so that we don't have to haul those feelings around with us forever, weighing us down."

— Elizabeth Gilbert

- Rituals acknowledge our most wonderful highs and our deepest lows. They create ways for us to assemble to celebrate life's joys and heal hurts that are beyond words. That's why we have birthday cake and candles, graduation ceremonies, weddings, and funerals, among many other rituals large and small.
- When you and your friend are grieving his cancer, you may each (separately or together) find the ritual of religious services soothing and meaningful. If you haven't attended for a while, try it again. Or try walking a labyrinth or meditating.
- You can create new ceremonies to mark the milestones in your friend's cancer journey. When she's finished her treatment, for example, you can bring her friends and family together to celebrate. Make it a ritual by gathering in a circle and having each person share something they love about your friend. Close by releasing sky lanterns, also called wish lanterns, into the night sky.
- Creating day-to-day rituals that support your friend can also be extremely helpful. For instance, you can text him each morning with a thought for the day. Or you can start getting together with him every Tuesday afternoon for lunch and an activity. Or you can make Sunday night your "always call John" night.

CARPE DIEM
Today, find a way to use ritual to help both yourself and your friend.

98.

LIVE WITH GRATITUDE AND
COUNT YOUR BLESSINGS

"Gratitude unlocks the fullness of life. It turns what we have into enough, and more. It turns denial into acceptance, chaos to order, confusion to clarity. It can turn a meal into a feast, a house into a home, a stranger into a friend."

— Melody Beattie

- When someone you care about is faced with a horrible disease like cancer, and you yourself feel pain as you witness the many losses, it can be difficult to maintain a sense of gratitude about life.

- Yet, as we've said, one message cancer patients have spoken to us loudly and clearly is that they want their loved ones to appreciate every moment of their own lives.

- Think of all that you have to be thankful for. This is not to minimize any hardships you may be experiencing at the moment but rather to allow you to reflect on the possibilities for love and joy each day. Honor those possibilities and have gratitude for them. Be grateful for your life and gifts. Be grateful for your family and friends. Above all, be grateful for this very moment. When you are grateful, you prepare the way for inner peace.

CARPE DIEM
Today, tell someone in the form of a written note or letter that you are grateful for them.

99.

BELIEVE IN YOUR CAPACITY TO HEAL AND GROW THROUGH GRIEF

"Don't go through life. Grow through life."
— Eric Butterworth

- In time, you may find that both you and your friend are growing emotionally and spiritually as a result of her cancer grief journey. Depending on where she is right now in her journey, she may not be ready to discuss or consider growth yet. But even if she's not ready, she can still believe that it's out there waiting for her. You too.
- Growth means a new inner balance with no end points. No, your life will never be exactly the same as it was before your loved one was diagnosed with cancer—but it might be more fulfilling.
- Growth means exploring our assumptions about life. Ultimately, exploring our assumptions about life after a brush with a life-threatening illness can make those assumptions richer and more life-affirming.
- Growth means using our potentials. The encounter with cancer reawakens us to the importance of using our potentials—our capacities to mourn our losses openly and without shame, to be interpersonally effective in our relationships with others, and to continue to discover fulfillment in life, living, and loving.

CARPE DIEM
Consider the ways in which you may be growing emotionally and spiritually since your friend's diagnosis.

100.

GIVE YOURSELF A HAND

"A kind gesture can reach a wound that only compassion can heal."
— Steve Maraboli

- Being a good friend during times of grief and loss is an art that few of us master.
- If you've been there for your friend with cancer, if you've been his companion through this most difficult of journeys, you are to be congratulated.
- It is the relationships in our lives that give life meaning. You have nurtured a loving relationship as well as helped another human being heal.
- Thank you for your empathy. Thank you for your compassion. The world needs more people like you.

CARPE DIEM
Treat yourself to something special you've been wanting to buy or do. You deserve it. As Eeyore said to Pooh, "You're a real friend."

OUR PRAYER FOR YOU

May the ideas in this book help activate your empathy and inspire you to become the best cancer companion you can be.

May you embrace and reap the rewards of giving the gift of your presence.

May you help your friend mourn so that she can live and love fully.

May you learn to mourn your own grief and accept support for yourself along the way.

May you find ways to persevere, even when you are busy and the going gets tough.

May you look for beauty even in the ugliest moments.

May you find hope when you need it.

May you nurture your own spirit in ways that bring you closer to your self and to God.

May you live with purpose and love each and every day of your life.

May you find untapped stores of compassion within yourself so that you can be kind to yourself as well as help others in need.

Blessings to you as you continue to explore your lessons learned, questions asked, and choices made.

We wish you peace and joy!

A Self-Companionship Manifesto for Cancer Companions

Those of us who companion others through illness and grief have a wondrous opportunity: to help others embrace and grow through their challenges—and to lead fuller, more deeply lived lives ourselves because of this experience.

But being a good cancer companion is draining—physically, emotionally, and spiritually. We must first care for ourselves if we want to care well for others. This manifesto is intended to empower you to practice good self-companionship along the way.

1. **I deserve to lead a joyful, whole life.**
    No matter how much I care (and worry) about the person who has cancer, my life is multifaceted. My family, my other friends, my interests, and my spirituality also deserve my time and attention. I deserve my time and attention.

2. **I am not the only one who can help the person who has cancer.**
    When I feel indispensable, I tend to ignore my own needs. There are others who can also provide companionship to my friend. I can reach out to them and ask them to join me in supporting her.

3. **I must maintain or develop healthy eating, sleeping, and exercise patterns.**
    I am aware of the importance of these things for my friend who has cancer, but I may neglect them myself. A well-balanced diet, adequate sleep, and regular exercise allow me to be the best I can be.

4. **I must maintain boundaries in my friendship with the person with cancer.**
    Of course I get emotionally involved, because that's what friends do. Active empathy allows me to be a good companion. However, I must always remember I am responsible *to* other adults, not *for* them.

5. **I am not perfect and I must not expect myself to be.**
I wish my helping efforts were always successful. But even when I offer compassionate, "on-target" help, the recipient of that help isn't always prepared to use it. And when I do make mistakes, I should see them as an integral part of learning and growth, not as measurements of my self-worth.

6. **I must practice effective time-management skills.**
I must set practical goals for how I spend my time. I must also remember Pareto's principle: twenty percent of what I do nets eighty percent of my results.

7. **I must also practice setting limits and alleviating stresses I can do something about.**
I must try to have reasonable goals and set realistic expectations of myself. I should enjoy what I do accomplish in helping my friend but shouldn't berate myself for what is beyond me.

8. **I must listen to my inner voice. As a cancer companion, I will at times become grief overloaded.**
When my inner voice begins to whisper its fatigue, I must listen carefully and allow myself some downtime.

9. **I must express the unique me. I shouldn't be afraid to companion using my unique talents and abilities.**
I must also make time each day to remind myself of what is important to me. If I only had three months to live, what would I do?

10. **I must remember that I am a spiritual being.**
I will spend alone time focusing on self-understanding and self-love. To be present to those I companion, I must appreciate the beauty of life and living. I must renew my spirit.

ALSO BY ALAN WOLFELT
AND KIRBY DUVALL

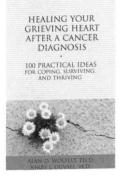

Healing Your Grieving Heart After a Cancer Diagnosis

100 Practical Ideas for Coping, Surviving, and Thriving

by Alan D. Wolfelt, Ph.D. and Kirby J. Duvall, M.D.

Being diagnosed with cancer is a major blow—physically, emotionally, socially, cognitively, and spiritually. All aspects of your self are under assault at the same time. And no matter the type or stage of cancer, the treatment plan, or the prognosis, your new and frightening grief can rattle you to your core. This book by Drs. Alan Wolfelt and Kirby Duvall will help you understand and cope with your many difficult thoughts and feelings and find ways to experience peace and joy in the journey. Some of the 100 ideas explain the basic principles of grief and mourning and how they apply to the life-altering, life-threatening, or terminal medical diagnosis. Others offer immediate, here-and-now suggestions of things you can do today to express your grief and live with meaning in each moment.

ISBN 978-1-61722-200-9 • 128 pages • softcover • $11.95

Companion
P R E S S

All Dr. Wolfelt's publications can be ordered by mail from
Companion Press
3735 Broken Bow Road
Fort Collins, CO 80526
(970) 226-6059
www.centerforloss.com

ALSO BY ALAN WOLFELT

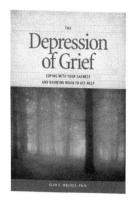

The Depression of Grief
Coping with Your Sadness and Knowing When to Get Help

When someone you love dies, it's normal and necessary to grieve. Grief is the thoughts and feelings you have inside you, and sadness is often the most prominent and painful emotion. In other words, it's normal to be depressed after a loss. This compassionate guide will help you understand your natural depression, express it in ways that will help you heal, and know when you may be experiencing a more severe or clinical depression that would be eased by professional treatment. A section for caregivers that explores the new DSM-5 criteria for Major Depression is also included.

"This enlightening book revealed to me that I am not flawed and it further gave me the strength to go back and do a bit more work so I could truly mourn the loss of my mom and start living life once again." — Kerry Bratton

"This is a much needed resource for both persons who are experiencing grief and professional caregivers who often have a limited understanding of the subtle differences between grief and clinical depression. This book is not only thorough and informative; it is written in a way that is relevant to any person involved in grief and bereavement work." — Jane Castle

ISBN 978-1-61722-193-4 • 128 pages • softcover • $14.95

Companion
PRESS

All Dr. Wolfelt's publications can be ordered by mail from
Companion Press
3735 Broken Bow Road
Fort Collins, CO 80526
(970) 226-6059
www.centerforloss.com

ALSO BY ALAN WOLFELT

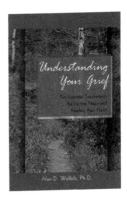

Understanding Your Grief

Ten Essential Touchstones for Finding Hope and Healing Your Heart

One of North America's leading grief educators, Dr. Alan Wolfelt has written many books about healing in grief. This book is his most comprehensive, covering the essential lessons that mourners have taught him in his three decades of working with the bereaved.

In compassionate, down-to-earth language, *Understanding Your Grief* describes ten touchstones—or trail markers—that are essential physical, emotional, cognitive, social, and spiritual signs for mourners to look for on their journey through grief.

The Ten Essential Touchstones:

1. Open to the presence of your loss.
2. Dispel misconceptions about grief.
3. Embrace the uniqueness of your grief.
4. Explore your feelings of loss.
5. Recognize you are not crazy.
6. Understand the six needs of mourning.
7. Nurture yourself.
8. Reach out for help.
9. Seek reconciliation, not resolution.
10. Appreciate your transformation.

Think of your grief as a wilderness—a vast, inhospitable forest. You must journey through this wilderness. To find your way out, you must become acquainted with its terrain and learn to follow the sometimes hard-to-find trail that leads to healing. In the wilderness of your grief, the touchstones are your trail markers. They are the signs that let you know you are on the right path. When you learn to identify and rely on the touchstones, you will find your way to hope and healing.

ISBN 978-1-879651-35-7 • 176 pages • softcover • $14.95

Companion
P R E S S

All Dr. Wolfelt's publications can be ordered by mail from
Companion Press
3735 Broken Bow Road
Fort Collins, CO 80526
(970) 226-6059
www.centerforloss.com

ALSO BY ALAN WOLFELT

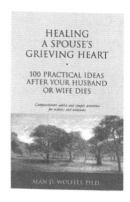

Healing a Spouse's Grieving Heart

100 Practical Ideas After Your Husband or Wife Dies

When your spouse dies, your loss is profound. Not only have you lost the companionship of someone you deeply loved, you have lost your helpmate, your lover, the person you shared your history, and perhaps your financial provider. Learning to cope with your grief and find continued meaning in life will be difficult, but you can and you will if you embrace the principles set down in this practical guide.

This book offers 100 practical, here-and-now suggestions for helping widows and widowers mourn well so they can go on to live well and love well again. Whether your spouse died recently or long ago, you will find comfort and healing in this compassionate book.

ISBN 978-1-879651-37-1 • 128 pages • softcover • $11.95

Companion
P R E S S

All Dr. Wolfelt's publications can be ordered by mail from
Companion Press
3735 Broken Bow Road
Fort Collins, CO 80526
(970) 226-6059
www.centerforloss.com

ALSO BY ALAN WOLFELT

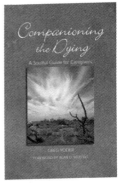

Companioning the Dying
A Soulful Guide for Caregivers
by Greg Yoder, Foreword by Alan D. Wolfelt

Based on the assumption that all dying experiences belong not to the caregivers but to those who are dying—and that there is no such thing as a "good death" or a "bad death" —*Companioning the Dying* helps readers bring a respectful, nonjudgmental presence to the dying while liberating them from self-imposed or popular expectations to say or do the right thing.

Written with candor and wit by hospice counselor Greg Yoder, who has companioned several hundred dying people and their families, *Companioning the Dying* exudes a compassion and a clarity that can only come from intimate work with the dying. The book teaches through real-life stories that will resonate with both experienced and clinical professionals as well as laypeople in the throes of caring for a dying loved one.

ISBN 978-1-61722-149-1 • 148 pages • softcover • $19.95

Companion
PRESS

All Dr. Wolfelt's publications can be ordered by mail from
Companion Press
3735 Broken Bow Road
Fort Collins, CO 80526
(970) 226-6059
www.centerforloss.com

Training and Speaking
Engagements

To contact Dr. Wolfelt about speaking engagements or training opportunities at his Center for Loss and Life Transition, email him at DrWolfelt@centerforloss.com.